ABC'S

OF PAIN RELIEF AND TREATMENT:

ADVANCES, BREAKTHROUGHS, AND CHOICES

ABC'S

OF PAIN RELIEF
AND TREATMENT:

ADVANCES, BREAKTHROUGHS, AND CHOICES

Dr. Tim Sams

iUniverse, Inc.
New York Lincoln Shanghai

ABC'S OF PAIN RELIEF AND TREATMENT: ADVANCES, BREAKTHROUGHS, AND CHOICES

iUniverse books may be ordered through booksellers or by contacting:

iUniverse
2021 Pine Lake Road, Suite 100
Lincoln, NE 68512
www.iuniverse.com
1-800-Authors (1-800-288-4677)

ISBN-13: 978-0-595-38280-4 (pbk)
ISBN-13: 978-0-595-82649-0 (ebk)
ISBN-10: 0-595-38280-0 (pbk)
ISBN-10: 0-595-82649-0 (ebk)

Printed in the United States of America

I dedicate this book to anyone who has been suffering from long-term pain and to the five thousand pain patients and their spouses and children who let me into their lives over the past decade. You have been my teachers and my mentors. I have battled for you and with you, but always in awe of you. You have my profound respect. Your courage, integrity, and perseverance inspire us all to become better people. May you find in these pages some peace and hope.

Contents

Acknowledgments

First and foremost, I would like to acknowledge my pain physician colleagues who have taught me, encouraged me, and inspired me over the years. In general order and according to how long I have worked with them, they include: Scott Stoney, M.D., John Gurskis, M.D., Jeffrey Olsen, M.D., Holly Sata, M.D., Steve Snyder, M.D., Carl Hess, M.D., Clifford Bernstein, M.D., Michael Lowenstein, M.D., Vernon Williams, M.D., Richard Paicius, M.D., Kenneth Grabow, M.D., Stephen Barkow, M.D., Andrew Merritt, M.D., Mark Wardenburg, D.C., Timothy Downing, M.D., Paul Coluzzi, M.D., Larry Ho, M.D., Standiford Helm, M.D., Timothy Lynch, M.D., and Afshin Gerayli, M.D. Thank you all.

I also acknowledge my behavioral medicine mentors: at The University of Michigan, James Papsdorf, Ph.D., and at Michigan State University, William Hinds, Ph.D., and Daniel Price, Ph.D. In my pain internship at the Long Beach VAMC, Richard Hanson, Ph.D. and Kenneth Gerber, Ph.D.were invaluable and supportive mentors and teachers.

Grateful acknowledgement is made to several others:

To Marylin Calzadilla, Ph.D., my partner in pain services for the past five years. But for her, my lengthy book-writing sabbatical would never have happened and neither would this book.

To Fay Enshaian, my biofeedback therapist and friend for the past fifteen years. Although I learned much of the science of pain management from the physicians listed above, I learned most of the art from her.

To Eola Force, Nanette Coleman, and Kitty Allen for numerous and varied tasks and support.

To Candace Sinclair, Carl Hess, M.D., George Ball and Doris Ball, Ph.D., for timely and valuable editing help.

And as always, a special acknowledgment to my beautiful and supportive wife, Lari Wenzel, Ph.D. Her multi-tasking skills amaze all the people who know her.

Preface: A Cold Day in Hell

Medieval torture on ghastly hooks. Knives flashing. Flesh tearing. Blood drowns agonized pleading. Scramble down, screaming. Run away. Fire choking. Run fast, faster. No. Can't. Slowing down. Slow…motion. Like quicksand. Trapped in terror. Can't escape. Chest burning. Can't breathe enough. Can't breathe. Can't. Like a vise. It hurts. Moaning. I hear moaning. I'm moaning. I'm dreaming. Wake up. Wake up. Wake up! Wake up!

Heart racing, head pounding, wild eyed scanning the bedroom, no knives, or quicksand. Breathe, breathe. Vise lets up a little. Pain bad. Burning. It's bad. It's a bad day. Pulsing. A bad day today. I can't afford a bad day. Throbbing. God doesn't care. It's a very bad pain day today. Aching. Good morning. You've got stuff to do.

I decide to get out of bed and eight to ten minutes later, I'm standing. Bad idea. I take some medicine and go back to bed for a few minutes. Get up. This time only three or four minutes and I'm standing. Shaky walking, but not using the walls, like last time. Legs feel like they're in cement. I try to go to the bathroom, nearly fall asleep on the pot, and then make my way to the kitchen. Coffee and reading the newspaper, exhausted, trying to ignore the thousand needles and the crawly things. It amazes me what people think is important. All that wasted energy. I can remember when I had energy like that.

The house is a mess. I'll clean it later. I promised to run some errands. Run? Hobble, limp, make it through. This car sucks. It's like a horse and wagon. Why has the weather been so bad lately—cold, dark, and rainy? What's that song line about the "cold hearted orb that steals the night, removes the colors from our sight; red is gray and yellow white?" Describes the weather and my mood. You know, I'd be able to park up front if I had a permit. Thanks for nuthin' doc. I hope household goods are near the door. These tile floors are wet and slippery. What were they thinking?

Can't find the kitchen supplies. Why isn't there an employee to help me? Bunch of kids standing around doing nothing. I find the manager and get some help. There's the supplies. Let's cash out and go.

Waiting in line. The volume's turned up on my pain; throbbing, pounding like the bass in this little gang-banger's car. Could they go any slower? Now an old woman counting out her change. Jesus Christ. Shifting my weight on my legs, sighs and small grunts, face drawn and tight. I'm afraid I won't make it. You can do this. Finally, it's my turn. I suggest they should have two open registers. The cashier frowns at me as the manager looks on and I see myself through their eyes—a frustrated, bitchy, middle-aged woman, who thinks she's too good to have to wait.

I want to scream, "That's not fair! You don't know me. This isn't me. The real me died when the pain was born. This is miserable me." I can almost hear my mom say, "You never get a second chance to make a first impression." My heart sinks as I consider all the people who have only met the miserable, bitchy me. I fight back tears walking to the car.

Compose myself in the driver's seat for a moment. I take more medicine with yesterday's Starbucks. Yuck. I realize I can't physically turn around far enough to see behind me and slowly back out, just hoping. Some dirty looks, but who gives a shit. Now I feel empty and numb. I get some drive-through lunch so I can stay in the car and then on to my doctor's appointment.

It's business as usual there. Patient number 666 here. Happy to fill out the forms for the 200th time. Doctor's only running a half hour behind. What a shock. Pretty, young staff complaining about their boyfriends and the patient before me. I want to shake them and yell, "It's not business as usual. I'm in agony over here and you're supposed to do something about it!" How did this happen? How did I become an angry patient everywhere I go? Why can't I just get my refills over the phone? Because they want more money, that's why. They sure don't spend it on furniture. These chairs are like sitting in church.

By the time I get to the inner sanctum, I can barely walk or bend. I lie down on the exam table afraid I won't be able to get up again. He comes in on a rush of air, hurried, distracted. Look up, doc; I'm not in the chart. I'm right here. We discuss the procedure I'm having tomorrow. I describe some new symptoms but I can tell he's not really listening. He mumbles something about the procedure helping with that and leaves the room. So far, I got nine minutes of his precious time.

I realize he's not coming back. The nurse has to help me off the exam table. I have an appointment with the pain psychologist in a few minutes, but I cancel. I'm suffering horribly now. He'll probably think I'm being noncompliant. He sees me and asks a few questions in the hallway about the procedure tomorrow. I'll call to schedule a follow-up. I need to get home.

Somehow, I make it to my driveway without killing anyone and all I can think about is the couch. I am done, spent, and miserable. I hurt so badly. I feel sweaty and nauseated. Couch. Sweet couch. Here come the spasms as I start to relax. I turn the TV on for background noise hoping desperately to nap and then the phone rings. It's my daughter. She tells me how important it is that I stay busy and that I get out of the house more. She tells me about a friend who had the same problem and saw this doctor in Houston who got rid of it. She'll get his name for me. And maybe I should try this new church by her house. For the nth time that day, I want to scream, but I don't.

Tossing and turning, I don't sleep, but the pain volume settles into a steady, faded roar that I can mostly deal with. I did stop going to church sometime after my pain started. I pretty much feel royally shafted by God. I married, raised a family, and worked my ass off. I don't deserve this. I don't want to think about what I'm supposed to learn from this. I know bad things happen to good people, but this is just wrong. The old anger wells up at that woman for causing my injury in the first place, but I push it away.

I can't remember if I took my pain medication two or three times already, but I take another dose so I can do some light chores before my husband comes home. I tidy up a few rooms a little and decide to tackle the dishes. Partway through, a dish starts to fall, and I grab it before it hits the floor. Horrific, rending, excruciating pain that makes me see stars. Bile burns the back of my throat and I choke back the urge to vomit. Slowly, I make my way to the couch. Breathe. Breathe. Oh my God, what did I do? I'm so tense; every muscle in my body has a charley horse. The tears come freely now.

I'm devastated. I can't seem to do the simplest things anymore. I'm getting worse; not better. I feel so alone, so utterly, completely alone. I'm lost in my own private hell of pain and doctors' appointments and trying to act as if I'm like everyone else. I feel like an alien, observing the rest of the world with this detached numbness that would become rage if I let it. I see it all so clearly now with true perspective and wisdom. Either you hurt or you don't. If you hurt, you're screwed. If you don't, shut up. Get over it. It's not as important as you think.

The waterfall slows and stops. I hurt a little less, but I am exhausted in a way that a good night's sleep wouldn't touch. I feel vulnerable, open, and raw—like a child facing the closet bogeyman. Inexplicably, I dose off for a few minutes, awakened by a far-off voice that moves closer.

"Honey, you fell asleep. Were you making dinner or should I order?"

Even I understand how this must look. Feeling like a zombie, I stagger through the messy house, splash some water on my face, and start to cook, something, anything, while looking at the half-washed dishes.

Over dinner, he's complaining bitterly about his boss and some new project. I can hear the words, but I have to struggle to put them together and make sense of the story. Knife, fork, and salt—pick them up, and set them down. You see, everything is normal. You can do this. How was my day? I squelch the urge to tear up again.

"It was okay. I hurt a little worse today. I tried to keep busy."

He says inquiringly that we are invited to a poolside barbecue with some friends this weekend.

I shrug and say, "I'll try."

He asks if the doctors are helping me and suggests that maybe he'll come to my next appointment.

I say, "That's fine," knowing it will never happen.

We sit in front of the TV and I can tell he'd like some stress-reduction sex, but he can tell it's not going to happen. We go through the hurt routine for the thousandth time. No guilt tonight. I sit and watch beautiful people doing beautiful things that I used to love and was good at. They take it all for granted. They don't know what they have, or that it could be taken away in a millisecond. Feeling abused and defeated, I trudge upstairs to bed, with an extra sleeper in my hand.

My meds kick in and as I begin to drift, I review some of the day's events and settle on the pain shrink for a moment. He asked if I was afraid I wouldn't wake up after the procedure tomorrow. He means well. He actually believes that because he read some books he understands me. But, he is really freakin' clueless. I'm not afraid I won't wake up tomorrow. I'm afraid I will.

Introduction

It does indeed feel like a cold day in your own private hell when you have persistent pain, and you are not alone. There are over a billion people worldwide with chronic pain, including eighty million in the United States. Among the millions of yearly visits to physicians, upwards of 60 percent are for painful conditions. As the baby boomers in the U.S. age, they are spending ever more money and time on health care and painful medical conditions.

People in pain don't want a cold, distant lecture from a doctor, family member, or book. My library contains the manuscripts of dozens of pain physicians and psychologists—dry, scholarly texts about pain coping or management that read like the brittle parchment of a Latin primer. People in pain want usable information from a caring, competent discussion, born of the same urgency and passion for pain relief that they feel.

This book is driven by passion and guided by a singular purpose. Every person in pain who reads this book will have less pain, forever. You will discover the hierarchy of advanced, "cutting edge" medical treatments that you should be receiving, and you will learn how to seize the best care from your doctors. You will explore breakthroughs in pain coping that produce a pain-resistant life. Then, you will map the choices that lead inevitably to pain relief and healthier activity.

For every medical condition, an algorithm should organize the process of diagnosis and the order of treatments. Over the past decade, consensus standards of care have evolved to evidence-based medicine. This clinical model requires that treatment decisions be based upon clear and convincing medical research that demonstrates a particular treatment is effective for a particular diagnosis. Increasingly, insurance companies are paying only for evidence-based treatments. This compels health care providers to be able to document the research evidence that supports recommended treatments.

Recently, an evidence-based algorithm was developed for the continuum of acute and chronic pain problems. It treats pain as a distinct medical condition, not merely a side effect of the original illness or injury. This algorithm was condensed by the World Health Organization (W.H.O.) into an eleven-step treatment hierarchy that includes multiple health care specialists—from surgeons and interventional physicians to acupuncturists and pain psychologists. The W.H.O. hierarchy establishes performance guidelines for physicians, psychologists, and even patients themselves to maximize treatment effectiveness.

Most doctors who treat patients in pain do not know the pain algorithm or hierarchy of treatments for pain. Some doctors aren't qualified by education or training to provide the various treatments, and are reluctant to acknowledge the benefits of those treatments that they do not perform. Other doctors simply want the flexibility to choose preferred treatments without being held accountable to the research evidence or "state-of-the-art." The vast majority of physicians do not know that referral to a pain psychologist for bio-behavioral treatment is one of the eleven steps in the pain algorithm.

Pain psychologists may teach patients about coping strategies, but they can be extremely reluctant to confront patients about their ongoing, unhealthy behaviors, especially when patients are not compliant with treatment or otherwise sabotage their own progress. Many psychologists are unwilling to risk losing patients, money, or readers by offending anyone. One way or another, in spite of extensive medical treatments, Internet access, and self-help books, people in pain continue to stumble their way in the dark, blind to why their pain is not getting better.

You need to learn much of what the medical and psychological community knows about pain and discusses daily in team conferences around the world. Pain relief recommendations are too important, and the stakes are too high for hidden agendas, gauzy diplomacy, or cowardice. If you are serious about pain relief and seeking usable information, you deserve an honest, forthright communication from an expert who respects your intelligence, and believes you will appreciate a little constructive criticism where appropriate.

Physicians and psychologists know that even if you have a single diagnosis, persistent pain is almost always a function of multiple sources of tissue damage, e.g., inflammation, muscle strain, tendon or ligament damage, spinal disc bulge or tear, scar tissue, nerve-based pain, and endorphin deficits, etc. These pain triggers, in combination, are referred to as "multi-factoral pain," and will require multiple treatment modalities over time. The evidence-based, eleven-step hierarchy of pain treatments was developed to ameliorate all the factors that increase your pain.

In this book, for the first time, you can learn which pain treatments are evidence-based and positioned in the W.H.O. hierarchy and which are not. You will explore the specific pain triggers that are most likely worsening your pain, and which treatments in the W.H.O hierarchy are most likely to relieve your particular pain.

You are taught how to assess your pain doctor's credentials and to evaluate his performance through every step of pain treatment. You will become skilled at negotiating with your doctor and selecting the most effective treatment options. You will discover the four stages in the process of chronic pain treatment and explore the options in your stage.

You will learn the most important lifestyle changes that will provide you with pain relief and increased physical, pleasurable, social, and productive activity. You are taught the vital importance of exercise in your rehabilitation, and how you can exercise without increasing pain. You are trained to employ efficient ergonomics and pain-relieving posture, gait, and body mechanics. You learn strategies for pacing, setting limits, dealing with friends and family, and relaxing through pain in forty-five seconds.

Perhaps most importantly, in this book you are challenged to assess yourself as a patient, and the manner in which you assist or impede your doctor in providing you with pain relief. You have the opportunity to evaluate how you may frustrate your doctor unnecessarily and compromise your credibility. You are taught to assess the extent to which you are unwittingly sabotaging your medical care, and the changes you can make in your behavior to maximize treatment gains. You are confronted with the environmental problems that can interfere with your motivation to function at your best, and thereby increase your pain.

I have been a health and pain psychologist for a quarter century. I have trained hundreds of medical and psychological interns, residents, and fellows in pain management through the University of California—Irvine, and the Long Beach V.A. Medical Center. I have given lectures to physicians from coast to coast. I have treated and supervised the treatment of over 8,000 patients with pain, and assessed over a thousand patients for surgical clearance, e.g., spinal fusion, gastric bypass, spinal cord stimulation, and indwelling narcotic infusion.

As the founder of Psychological Advances in Coping Education (P.A.C.E., Inc.), I oversee a staff of pain psychologists and biofeedback therapists, and I have offices throughout Southern California. Our professional mission is to alleviate pain and improve health and quality of life.

I have learned that chronic pain is an immensely powerful, purposeful, and passionate adversary. It devours joy, initiative, and wonder. It strives to make you more motivated by fear than accomplishment, and more by avoiding pain than attaining goals. It is zealous in capturing your attention and then saying, "I'll let you know when you can have it back."

To win the battle against chronic pain, it takes an equal amount of power, purpose, and passion. If you are exhausted by the fight, your medical and psychological providers had better step up. Victory requires honesty, courage, planning, and perseverance by you and your doctors. It takes teamwork, trust, and mutual competence.

This book is alternatingly blunt and cajoling, deadly serious and humorous, technical and poetic. It was written to transcend your pain and re-capture your attention. It is not a diplomatically correct, feel good book that is meant to be read casually and tossed aside. It is meant to be lived. If you have only mild or occasional discomfort, and are looking for a cursory review of medical treatments, this is not your best source. However, if you have significant pain that is affecting your life, and you want to know the hierarchy of medical treatments, if you wish to extract the best care from your doctors, and you are willing to change selected behaviors to have less pain, this is the first book written for you. If you have loved ones in pain, you can digest the contents of this book, understand that they are responsible for their pain, and persuade them to read your copy of this book. Better yet, make them buy their own copy.

Though this book is encouraging and supportive, you will be taking a long hard look at yourself, your family, friends, and your doctors. Right here, right now, what you do to help yourself is more important than what anyone else does to help you. That may be a frightening reality, but therein lies a measure of control and hope.

May you come to understand that improved quality of life is inevitable if you follow the advances and breakthroughs in your Personal Pain Paradigm. The secret of pain relief is revealed in a few simple choices.

We have several hundred pages to relieve your pain forever. Let's get started.

1

The Accepted Hierarchy of Pain Treatments

They brought my new consult in on a gurney by private ambulance. From the waiting room I could hear her moaning and pleading for "a pain shot." The physicians were nonplused by this behavior but my heart rate picked up a little. They wheeled her into my office lying on her back with her eyes closed and her fists clenched. I asked the attendants to move her into one of the chairs. She complained bitterly that it would hurt her and she cursed loudly as they lifted her from the gurney and carried her to a chair.

She sat sobbing and staring straight at the floor. She began to hyperventilate, and she kept asking if she was getting a pain shot. I introduced myself and told her that she would not be receiving an injection today, but I assured her that she would be able to leave in thirty minutes if we could finish her intake interview quickly. I taught her a short breathing exercise. I then asked her to lift her right forefinger anytime she felt she needed to moan or was about to hyperventilate, and we would stop and do the breathing exercise.

Rhia was a 48-year-old Welsh, divorced female with a thirteen-year history of chronic low back pain who was status post three lumbar surgeries including spinal fusion from L3-S1 with hardware and iliac crest grafting. She lived in her own apartment but had 24-hour nursing care. She had spent twenty-three hours of each day in bed for the past year and a half. She was profoundly depressed and had been admitted to a psychiatric facility twice in the past year for attempted suicides. She was taking eleven medications, including psychotropics and twenty Vicodin a day. She was a recovering alcoholic with seventeen years of sobriety but smoked two packs a day. She had no friends, and was estranged from her adult children.

We only had to do the breathing exercise twice. Rhia calmed down and answered my questions, still staring at the floor, obviously angry, frustrated, and immensely sad. After obtaining her history (with five minutes to spare of our thirty-minute target), I explained the integrated medical and behavioral program with the latter referred to as Psychological Advances in Coping Education (PACE). This integrated treatment included medical interventions, aqua therapy, physical therapy, biofeedback, pain classes, individual behavior modification, assertion training, and cognitive reframing over the next month. Rhia reiterated several times that she did not want to complete this program. She did not want to work with us. We had nothing to offer her. I still asked her to try it.

Obviously, we had not established much rapport and I wanted to try to reach her, to get past all her anger and the walls. As she was getting ready to leave, I asked her what had changed for her. What was different? If she had one wish, what would it be?

For the first time, she showed an extra spark. She pulled herself up in her chair, looked me straight in the eyes, and said, "I want to die."

◆   ◆   ◆

Where do you start with a patient like Rhia, or any patient with pain for that matter? Are there physician guidelines for diagnoses and treatment? If so, are these guidelines standardized? Should all doctors who treat pain be following the same guidelines? Can patients learn to evaluate their doctor's treatment and know if they are getting good care? The answer to all these questions is yes.

In the simplest terms, a hierarchy of treatments exists for which there is medical documentation of effectiveness. You can learn and insist upon receiving the treatments in this hierarchy. You can also learn an integrated coping strategy to decrease pain. Finally, you can overcome the barriers to effective medical treatment you may erect. In sum, you can learn what your doctors can do for you; what you can do for you; and what you can do for your doctor. When you integrate these three approaches into practice, it is referred to as your Personal Pain Paradigm, and it forms the basis for effective living with pain.

WHAT IS THE HIERARCHY OF PAIN TREATMENTS DEVELOPED BY THE WORLD HEALTH ORGANIZATION?

The World Health Organization (W.H.O.) has established a generally accepted, worldwide hierarchy or ladder of treatments for pain. Generally, these treatments have been documented by medical research to be effective for at least some painful conditions. The lower a treatment is on the ladder, the more conservative the treatment, as measured by cost, likely side effects, and physical invasiveness. The higher a treatment is on the ladder, the fewer number of people are likely to benefit, and the treatment becomes more powerful and risky. In this context, the treatment ladder is like a pyramid that successively narrows the number of potential patients as you move up. As a rule, doctors should begin treatment of each pain patient with the lowest appropriate rungs of treatment and work their way to the top to maximize pain relief and quality of life. The ladder is presented below with the lower rungs at the bottom left and higher rungs at the top right.

Nerve ablation

Implanted Pumps

Spinal stimulation

Surgery

Behavioral treatments

Nerve blocks and other injections

Narcotics and other oral analgesics

Muscle relaxants

Physical and occupational therapy, Chiropractic, Acupuncture

Non-steroidal anti-inflammatories

Over-the-counter medications

What Are the Eleven Rungs on the W.H.O. Ladder Of Pain Treatments?

The first and lowest rung on the ladder is treatment with over-the-counter medications. For pain relief, these medications include simple analgesics like Tylenol, and anti-inflammatories such as aspirin, naproxen, and Ibuprofen. You may also benefit from various heating rubs or anesthetic creams. These medicinal preparations can provide excellent pain relief for various types of pain, from headache or stomach pain to musculoskeletal pain. We can also include certain nutritional supplements like glocosamine or other natural herbs or remedies that have medicinal properties. Some of these supplements may have powerful effects on pain and rehabilitation. Over-the-counter remedies can be very beneficial for both short-and long-term pain.

The second rung on the ladder is treatment with the prescription, non-steroidal anti-inflammatories (NSAIDs) such as Celebrex. These medications reduce inflammation by interfering with the body's natural inflammatory response to injury. They are considered stronger or riskier than the over-the-counter medications. They are much more expensive and may cause greater stomach upset. Many patients obtain effective pain relief from these NSAIDs.

The next rung of pain treatments on the W.H.O. ladder is the traditional therapeutic modality. Physical therapy, occupational therapy, aqua therapy, chiropractic, and acupuncture are basic therapeutic modalities. These treatments may involve passive care that is done for you, such as heat or massage, and active treatments that you perform yourself, like stretching. These treatments are much more expensive and time consuming than simple medications, and suggest a greater potential for negative side effects. Generally, all of the modalities except acupuncture were designed to rehabilitate musculoskeletal injuries or related conditions such as heart attack or stroke.

The fourth level of treatment is the use of muscle relaxants such as Flexeril, (Cyclobenzaprine), or Zanaflex (Tizanidine). These medications have a much greater potential for abuse and dependence than the previous medications and can cause death upon overdose. They are powerful drugs with global side effects that may include lethargy and mental confusion. They can also provide almost miraculous relief of severe muscle pain and help you get a wonderfully good night's sleep.

The fifth rung on the W.H.O. ladder includes treatment with even stronger oral analgesics than previously mentioned. Most common are the oral narcotics or opioids that are related chemically to the opium poppy and include drugs like Darvon (propoxyphene), Vicodin (Hydrocodone), OxyContin (continuous release Oxycodone hydrochloride), and Dilaudid (hydromorphone). Powerful oral steroids like the Medrol Dose Pack (Methylprednisolone) are also included in this category. Oral steroids may be used with acute, severe pain, especially immediately following injury. Steroids for pain are prescribed only for the short-term and usually through a descending dose over a period of about five days.

Finally, this fifth rung of analgesics includes oral headache medications such as Imitrex (Sumatriptan) or Maxalt (Rizotriptan).

Unlike anti-inflammatories or muscle relaxants, narcotics do not attempt to treat the source of the pain, but simply mask pain signals. Both narcotics and steroids are very powerful and produce central nervous system side effects with extreme potential for abuse and dependence. Thus, they are most effective for short-lived pain.

The sixth rung on the W.H.O. ladder involves treatment with non-emergency injections for localized pain relief or diagnosis. These injections include epidural steroid injections, selective nerve root blocks, stellate ganglion blocks, bier blocks, nerve injections into other body parts, trigger point injections, Botox injections, and Synvisc injections, etc. This treatment rung may involve diagnostic injections performed mainly, or solely, for the purpose of diagnosis, such as discogram, injecting dye as a marker, or facet joint injections.

Behavioral and psychological programs are on the seventh rung of the W.H.O. pain treatment ladder. Competent behavioral pain services should include biofeedback training for posture, gait, and body mechanics; classes in pain coping and rehabilitation; relaxation training; individual psychoeducation; and family education. Patients should also learn strategies for stress inoculation and management. Typically, a specially trained pain psychologist and a biofeedback therapist provide these services.

Surgery, the eighth rung on the W.H.O. ladder of treatment, is considered when the previous seven options either have failed, or were inappropriate. In this context, I am referring to surgery for the primary purpose of pain reduction. This might be the case, for example, for someone who has a small bulging disc in the lower back with associated gradual onset of low back pain, with no other symptoms. Surgical candidacy is somewhat equivocal, non-emergent, and solely for the purpose of pain relief, when the body's integrity and functional capacity has been essentially maintained.

Contrast the above non-emergent, equivocal candidate with the patient who has immediate onset of neck pain following an accident. There is an eleven millimeter herniated disc in the neck that is compressing the spinal cord with associated numbness and loss of motor function in both arms. This patient is at risk for at least partial, permanent loss of arm and hand function or even quadriplegia. The risks of delaying surgery may outweigh any potential benefits from more conservative W.H.O. pain treatments. This patient needs at least disc compression surgery, probably immediately, independent of the potential for pain relief. In this case, the primary goal of surgery is not pain relief, but avoidance of paralysis and improvement in arm and hand function. Pain relief is a desired, if secondary, effect of surgery.

The ninth rung on the W.H.O. ladder of pain treatments is neuromodulation—most commonly by use of the spinal cord stimulator, also called the dorsal column stimulator. This implantable device provides pain relief by electrically stimulating the painful area to block pain perception. Like narcotics, the spinal cord stimulator works by masking the pain signal, not by treating the underlying condition. With spinal cord stimulation, electrical leads are implanted in the epidural space of the spine. The leads are often attached to the nerve roots that exit the spine and travel down the arms or legs. A generator or battery unit is also implanted with wires that connect to the electrical leads. The spinal cord stimulator transmits electrical energy that produces a sensation of warm vibration in the painful area that effectively masks the pain.

Like narcotics, spinal cord stimulation rarely provides 100 percent pain relief, but can provide 50 percent or greater pain relief, most often in the arms or legs. A trial period of stimulation is usually conducted for a week. The leads are placed through incisions at the spine but wires run externally to a generator that is worn in a pack around the waist. Thus, a patient is able to assess, in a variety of different situations, how much pain relief the stimulator will provide if the leads and the generator are permanently implanted. For patients who are good stimulator candidates, this treatment can provide excellent, almost instantaneous relief. Most board certified pain physicians can provide this treatment or refer you to someone who can.

The tenth rung on the W.H.O. ladder, and the final rung for most pain patients is the use of an indwelling infusion pump. It is an implanted device, similar to a spinal cord stimulator, which uses liquid medication rather than electrical stimulation to provide pain relief. A hockey puck-sized metal reservoir and combination battery-driven pump are implanted in the abdomen with a catheter that sends medicine, usually a narcotic, into the cerebral spinal fluid, typically in the low back. The medicine is absorbed by spinal tissue and acts upon pain receptors in the spinal cord.

Unlike oral narcotics, the indwelling infusion pump does not provide centralized, total-body pain relief. An oral narcotic courses throughout the bloodstream and produces a circulating blood level of medication that will decrease pain in almost any injured body part such as a burned hand, a broken leg, a pulled groin muscle, or a headache. Because the medicine from the infusion catheter is pumped directly into the spine, it does not course throughout the blood stream.

Rather than total body pain relief, the pump provides pain relief only in the low back or legs.

However, if the patient only has low back or leg pain, the lack of circulating narcotic provides several benefits. There is no burden on the liver and kidneys to metabolize or excrete the medication. There are virtually no brain-based side effects like lethargy or mental confusion. A much lower dose can be used than is the case for oral narcotics (1/300th) and the dose can be titrated (increased) with less concern for side effects. The pump provides a perfectly level dose of medication without the highs and lows that are almost inevitable with oral narcotics. Perhaps most importantly, more medication reaches the receptors in the low back that are actually sending pain signals. This can result in much more complete pain relief.

The eleventh and final pain treatment on the W.H.O. ladder is neurosurgical ablation. With this treatment, neurosurgeons attempt to destroy or cut the nerves that are sending pain signals. This can be done centrally by destroying a portion of the brain, or more peripherally by severing or destroying nerves that enervate the painful body part. This treatment was much more common twenty to thirty years ago when there were fewer treatment options available. As with most pain conditions, especially spine pain that radiates into the arms or legs, this is a highly risky treatment, with side effects that are essentially irreversible, and may include increased pain, loss of motor function, or paralysis. Almost none of the physicians that I have worked with over the years support this type of treatment in its original form.

In the past decade, however, there has been a resurgence of certain types of neuroablation where the risks are much lower. It is a reasonable treatment option for patients with severe, unremitting "phantom limb" pain following amputation. Many pain physicians provide neurosurgical ablations through radiofrequency of the small nerves associated with pain in the facet joints of the spine. Ablation may also be attempted for pain relief with some of the small nerves in the head, hands, or feet.

How Is the W.H.O. Ladder of Pain Treatments Used?

How is the W.H.O. ladder of pain treatments actually used in clinical practice? It varies widely from doctor to doctor. The above treatments are merely guidelines with no hard and fast, rigid criteria. Typically, each treatment is tried in succession for a period of days or months until it is deemed a success or failure in either eliminating or adequately decreasing the pain. If the treatment is successful in achieving permanent pain relief, treatment is terminated. If a treatment level or type is not successful in pain elimination, you and your doctor may decide to proceed to the next level.

Your doctor may eventually reach the conclusion that your pain is unlikely to go away completely or in the near future. This determination may be made because you have a progressive injury or disease, because your body is so severely damaged, or because you have suffered with pain for so long that medical treatment cannot provide complete healing and freedom from pain. Once such a determination has been made, the treatment goal shifts from pain cure to pain reduction and improved function. Therefore, you may be satisfied with maintaining a treatment level that provides impressive, if incomplete, pain relief. Whether or not you should advance to the next rung on the W.H.O. ladder then becomes a subjective decision. The success or failure of a given treatment level is assessed by you and your doctor, based in part on your respective expectations and goals. Ultimately, the two of you will decide whether you have achieved sufficient pain relief to warrant maintaining a treatment level and not ascending to the next level.

Your credibility with your doctor and the quality of the patient-doctor relationship will have a huge impact on this subjective decision. The key point is that the maintenance or escalation of treatment level is a mutual decision between you and your doctor. The doctor cannot force you to proceed with a new treatment that you refuse to accept, and you cannot force a doctor to prescribe a treatment that he refuses. In either of these circumstances, he may terminate you as a patient and you may find another doctor. Some patients do not understand that a doctor has the right to terminate their care, and they have the right to choose another doctor. Always.

If the mutual decision is made that a specific level of treatment does not adequately decrease your pain, you and your doctor can proceed to the next level. Then you will repeat the process of treatment and decision-making about an adequately successful outcome at the higher level. This process will happen repeatedly if you work your way up the ladder of treatments.

Throughout this process, it is critical to ensure that the treatment goals and expectations held by you and your doctor are clearly delineated and as similar as possible. If your doctor's treatment goal is to decrease your pain by 50 percent and yours is to be pain free enough to be able to perform all of your typical activities, then he may be much more conservative in moving you up the treatment ladder. This is a very common situation, especially with people who have very physically active lifestyles or high-paying, physically demanding employment.

Common sense tells us that by the time a doctor is involved, the patient has probably already tried over-the-counter remedies that have failed. At the initial consultation, your doctor may recommend several levels of treatment, simultaneously, in the belief that multiple levels are necessary for maximally beneficial medical care. For example, you might go to your doctor with a rapid onset of low back pain after shoveling snow and be diagnosed with low back strain. Your doctor might prescribe a combination of an anti-inflammatory, a short course of physical therapy, and a muscle relaxant as needed.

WHAT ARE THE MEDICAL SPECIALTIES THAT TREAT PAIN?

Primary care doctors, including family practice and internal medicine, manage the majority of new onset pain complaints. Chiropractic doctors are frequently consulted for new onset of orthopedic or neuromuscular pains. These doctors will prescribe various levels of pain treatment within their scope of practice. Following a process of diagnosis and treatment, they may decide to refer you to a specialist, such as an orthopedist, neurosurgeon, neurologist, cardiologist, podiatrist, or gastroenterologist. There are no absolute criteria for when to make these referrals. Like any specialist, physicians who specialize in the treatment of pain receive referrals from other physicians, most commonly primary care doctors, or surgeons.

In the context of the W.H.O. ladder of pain treatments, referrals to a specialist are most often made when the doctor is considering moving you up to a higher level of treatment on the ladder. This can happen when surgery is an option, injections are being considered, or when the patient may benefit from narcotics or much stronger narcotics than the referring physician is comfortable prescribing. In this situation, the referring doctor may maintain primary pain treating status or hand off your pain treatment entirely to the new doctor. Treatment is more commonly transferred when the referral is to a pain physician. You should know what your doctor's intentions are regarding continuing care when he refers you to another provider.

Pain medicine has become a medical specialty over the past twenty years with board certification recognizing specialty education, fellowship training, and passing a national test.

In a personal communication, my colleague Carl Hess, M.D. stated that, "Much of society doesn't really believe in long-term pain or believes that it is being over treated. This ignorance extends from government, doctors, and nurses to the family and friends of people in pain. This is a tragic barrier to effective pain treatment and control. People in pain should always have access to an educated and specialized treatment regimen using the most advanced and powerful pain relieving techniques available" (2005).

Board certified pain physicians are experts in the W.H.O. ladder and will provide or oversee the various pain treatments. As you move up the ladder, the treatments require input from many different disciplines or specialists such as a physical therapist, acupuncturist, chiropractor, pain psychologist, or surgeon. Your doctor may integrate several treatment levels or disciplines into your care. Hundreds of research studies have demonstrated that a combined treatment approach is more effective for long-term pain than any single treatment. Thus, the most effective treatment for pain is referred to as "multi-disciplinary."

Pain physicians often establish integrated pain centers that can provide most or all of the disciplines and treatments in a central facility. This is more convenient for the patient and facilitates communication between the various providers. You may be able to receive medications, injections, physical therapy, acupuncture, behavioral services, and even implantable devices at the same location. At a pain center, the providers from each discipline meet in formalized team conferences to discuss your care and to plan each step in your treatment. A partial list of pain clinics in the United States is available at my Web site: www. MyPainReliefDoc.com/pain-clinics.htm, or upon written request to Dr. Tim Sams, c/o PACE, Inc., P.O. Box 6599, Irvine, CA, 92616.

MOVING BETWEEN RUNGS ON THE W.H.O. LADDER

Frequently, a doctor who evaluates you upon referral may decide to try levels of treatment that were provided to you previously and considered failures. This is perfectly acceptable practice. Your doctor may want to try a different medication or type of injection. You might undergo spine surgery through a microdiscectomy, then require a laminectomy the next year, and a spinal fusion the following year. You might receive additional spinal injections that were ineffective before surgery, but might provide pain relief for post-surgical, residual pain.

With long-term pain, you might be maintained on a regimen that includes several injections a year indefinitely. Or, you might receive many courses of physical therapy over the years for severe flare-ups of long-term pain. The point is that you do not necessarily finish forever with one level of treatment simply because you have progressed to the next level. You may move up and down the ladder as new treatments become available or as ongoing treatments become less effective.

You can and should use your new knowledge about the W.H.O. pain treatment ladder to evaluate the care you are receiving from the doctor treating your pain problem. If your pain level is unacceptable, you should suggest that your doctor consider the next treatment level on the ladder. If your doctor cannot or will not provide that level of treatment, you should discuss the reasoning and determine how you wish to proceed.

Chiropractors cannot prescribe narcotics. Internists cannot perform major surgery. Many family practice physicians will not write scripts for the stronger, continuous-release narcotics. Therefore, it may be in your best interests to request a referral to someone who can and will provide a higher level of treatment. At a minimum, you may pursue a consultation with a second opinion doctor about your candidacy for the higher treatment level. If your pain has existed for more than one year, you may want to request a referral to a Board Certified pain physician whose entire career is dedicated to pain relief.

This is your life, your body, and your pain. Your doctor is not your friend. She is a paid service vendor and a highly paid one at that. You should ask for what you want and do not be shy.

Living well with passion and purpose in spite of pain requires the knowledge that, "I can do this." I can change my pain and myself. I can make life meaningful and even joyful.

At the end of each chapter, we will summarize the critical, healthy changes as ICAN.

I can use the W.H.O. ladder to improve my medical pain care

Insight—The W.H.O. ladder should guide my pain treatment.

Commitment—I will study the W.H.O. ladder as it relates to my past and present pain treatment.

Action—I will discuss my pain treatment plan with my doctor from the W.H.O. ladder perspective.

Now—I will maintain a medical information journal called, "Taking Aim Against Pain (TAAP)" and write my W.H.O. ladder questions in it for my next doctor's appointment. I will use a standard ring binder, or download a custom-

ized TAAP journal at www.MyPainReliefDoc.com. Or, to receive a TAAP journal through the mail, I will call 877-545-7272.

2

The Basics of Pain Transmission and Sensitization

You have learned the general hierarchy of treatment types for pain. Now we discuss how your pain doctor conceptualizes your pain and how that should affect the specific treatment decisions she makes. To evaluate the quality of your pain care, you need to understand the different diagnostic categories of pain that should determine your treatment and the basic mechanisms of pain transmission. This chapter contains a fair amount of medical and physiological information that can be tough reading when you hurt. However, it explains the reasoning behind and the critical importance of the strategies in the subsequent chapters. I will be brief, but, first, I need you to complete an exercise.

I would like you to get a pencil or pen right now. Get up if you need to and then come back. This is where you show your motivation and integrity. I'll wait, patiently.

Settled in? Okay. In the space below, I want you to describe your pain in so much detail that anyone reading the paper would know in their heart what your pain is really like for you. Use as many sentences, phrases, or words as you can. Don't stop until you've written twelve or thirteen lines' worth of incredibly detailed description. This is your chance to communicate honestly, without censoring anything, and to explain exactly what your pain is like in all its terrible suffering. If you get stuck, you might think about the story in the Preface of this book, *A Cold Day in Hell*, and any parts with which you can identify. Once again, do you just want to read about pain, or do you want to learn how to decrease it? The choice is yours. Let yourself go as you describe your pain and miserable suffering. I will be here when you get back.

My pain is: _____

_____

_____

_____

_____

_____

_____

_____

_____

_____

_____

_____

_____

_____

_____

A Summary of the Nervous System

Welcome back. What was that like? Do you think people would be surprised by what you wrote? Do you think your family would understand? Are there things on the paper that make you uncomfortable? Let's just sit with your pain description and we will return to what you have written in a few chapters.

Pain is a function of your nervous system, a living biochemical electrical circuit, the fundamental unit of which is called a nerve cell or neuron. The most common type of neuron is roughly shaped like your hand and arm from fingernails to elbow. The fingers of the neuron (dendrites) receive an electrical signal from an adjacent nerve that can actually be measured in millivolts of electricity. These signals are transmitted across the hand (cell body) to the arm (axon). If the electrical signal from the hand, (cell body) is strong enough where it joins the arm at the wrist (axon hillock), a signal will travel all the way down the arm (axon) to the end at your elbow (axon terminal). The axon terminal is connected to one of the dendrites of the next neuron which receives the electrical signal and then transmits the signal down that neuron to the next one; a process that may be repeated across thousands of neurons in rapid succession.

Anatomically, your nerves are divided into the central and peripheral nervous systems. The central nervous system is comprised of nerves in the brain and the spinal cord. The peripheral nervous system is comprised of all other nerves. The spinal cord sends nerve bundles out on the left and right sides at each vertebra. In the neck or cervical area of the spine, these nerve bundles extend from your spinal cord down to your hands. In the mid torso or thoracic area, the nerve bundles extend from your spinal cord around your torso into your chest and abdomen. In the low back or lumbar area, the nerve bundles extend from your spinal cord down to your feet.

WHAT ARE THE PAIN PATHWAYS IN THE HUMAN BODY?

Different types and locations of nerves have different functions. Some nerves help us experience our environment through taste, touch, sight, sound, or smell. Some help us walk and bend and move around. And some sense pain. When you stub your toe, the "ouch" travels like a telephone wire up your toe to your foot, ankle, leg, thigh, and then into the lumbar spinal cord where it travels up your spine and is received by your brain. When you burn your hand, the call goes up your hand, arm, shoulder, and into the cervical spinal cord and then up into your brain. Thus, there is a pathway made of adjacent, sequential neurons, that must fire in rapid succession from peripheral nerves in the feet or hands to central nerves in the spinal cord and then up to the brain where the electrical message is interpreted as pain. Ultimately, all pain is in the brain. What does not reach the brain is not pain.

Painful sensory input from an event like a stubbed toe is picked up by nerve endings or pain receptors in your toe and foot and transmitted via different sets of nerve pain fibers to nerve cells in the lumbar spine and then up to the brain. This pathway is known as the ascending tract. There are three main ascending nerve pain fibers of different sizes, speeds, and composition. The first fiber is the A-Beta nerve fiber composed of large neurons heavily covered with a sheath called myelin. This sheath causes A-Beta fibers to transmit pain signals very quickly. This fast pain, referred to as primary pain, is usually experienced as pressure.

The second nerve fibers are A-Delta fibers, which are smaller than A-Beta fibers and slower since they have less myelin sheath to speed transmission. A-Delta pain tends to feel sharp or stabbing. The third nerve fibers are C fibers, which are also smaller than A-Beta fibers and even slower than A-Delta since they have no myelin sheath to speed the signal. C fiber pain is perceived as burning or the all-too-familiar dull, aching, or cramping pain. The slower A-Delta and C fiber pain is also called secondary pain. Pain from the slower A-Delta and C fibers is almost always perceived as more severe than pain from the faster A-Beta fibers.

All three types of nerve fibers send painful messages up the spinal cord to the lowest part of the brain, which is the relay station, called the brain stem. However, once there, the fast A-Beta fibers follow the neospinothalamic path and terminate at brain structures called the thalamus and cortex. Interestingly, the cortex is where most high-level thinking and reasoning happens. The slower A-Delta and C fibers follow the paleospinothalamic path and terminate at the hypothalamus and limbic structures; the latter of which is responsible for processing emotional responses and feelings. This means that <u>the same brain structures responsible for thoughts and feelings are also responsible for pain perception</u>.

Human brains are constantly being bombarded with thousands of sensations per second, both internally produced and externally perceived through the five senses. The brain needs a way to sift rapidly through both painful and non-painful stimuli and prioritize them in terms of what needs the most attention and action.

THE GATE CONTROL THEORY OF PAIN

The Gate Control Theory of pain was first developed in the 1960s by Ronald Melzack, Ph.D., and Patrick Wall, M.D., in part to explain how the body prioritizes pain. It recognized that how much pain you experience from a particular painful stimulus is determined not just by the intensity of the stimulus but by other factors, too. These other factors often reflect the brain's way of prioritizing the importance of the pain. For instance, a gradually increasing painful stimulus is often perceived as less painful than a stimulus that is suddenly applied even when they reach the same level of stimulation.

Years ago, eight-year-old boys taught scientists that frogs placed in water, which was slowly heated to boiling, would not try to jump out before they perished. With the gradual increase in discomfort, their brains simply did not make pain a priority. You may have had similar experiences with gradually increasing pain even without the boiling water.

The Gate Control Theory maintains that biochemical and physiological changes in the nervous system can either open the gates to make perceived pain worse, or close gates to make pain less severe. Subsequent research demonstrated how these gates work. That research, in turn, led to more effective pain treatments.

Sequences of adjacent nerves may seem to function like telephone wires transmitting information from point A (peripheral nerves) to point B (the brain). However, on closer examination, each nerve looks more like a big tree trunk that extends downward with multiple levels of successively smaller roots connected to multiple sites in the ground.

Like a root system, a single nerve can have many hundreds of dendrites that are connected to hundreds of other sites (nerves) and receive information from all of these other nerves simultaneously. Some nerves connected to the dendrites provide excitatory impulses that encourage the nerve to transmit an electrical signal down its entire length and then to other cells. Some nerves connected to the dendrites send impulses that inhibit "firing" or discourage transmitting the electrical signal all the way down the axon. From a pain perspective, some of these connected nerves try to open pain gates and some try to close pain gates.

Nerve cells that can transmit pain messages continually receive a complex biochemical flux of both excitatory and inhibitory pain impulses from nearby nerves. An individual nerve cell will pass on the pain signal to other nerves when the excitatory impulses it is receiving are sufficiently greater than the inhibitory impulses. Once the excitatory threshold is reached, the pain message is transmitted from one end of the nerve cell to the other end, and out to adjacent cells.

Peripheral nerves send nerve fibers up the spinal cord and into the brain. These ascending nerve fibers mainly send excitatory information from peripheral nerves to the spinal cord. From a Gate Control perspective, these ascending nerve fibers open pain gates. However, there are also inhibitory signals in the spinal cord, acting on each of the nerve fibers to encourage the pain gates to close. If the inhibitory signals are sufficiently strong across all of the nerve fibers, all of the pain gates will close. Since the pain signal does not reach the brain, the sensation of pain is eliminated. This is what happens with a spinal block during labor and delivery. Certainly, excitatory pain messages are being sent by the pelvic area, but they are overwhelmed by the much more powerful inhibitory messages coming from the anesthetic agents in the spinal block at the level of the spinal cord. Going back to our tree analogy, the roots cannot communicate with the leaves if the trunk is cut in half.

With many pain-relieving treatments, however, not all of the nerve fibers are prevented from sending the pain signal. Some nerve fibers receive more excitatory impulses than inhibitory ones, so some of the pain gates remain open. In these situations, there will only be pain reduction and not elimination since some of the pain signals will still reach the brain. This often occurs with oral narcotics after surgery; pain is decreased but not eliminated.

Immediately after an injury, the A-Beta nerve fibers "light up" and open the pain gates for fast pressure pain signals. Within a few seconds, the slower A-Delta and C fibers begin to "light up" and open the pain gates for a sharp and stabbing or aching, burning pain sensation. The excitation of these slower fibers inhibits the signal from the fast A-Beta fibers that closes their pain gates. The pressure sensation of the fast fibers is thus replaced by one or more different painful sensations from the slow fibers. However, the slower A-Delta and C fibers also compete with each other. Strong excitation of one set of pain fibers is associated with inhibition of the other set at the level of the spinal cord.

One example of this competition between the different types of nerve fibers happens when you whack your shin on the coffee table in the dark. The fast A-Beta pressure sensation lasts only a second and is replaced by a sharp pain and then throbbing, aching pain as the A-Delta fibers kick in, followed next by the C fibers. You may have found that rubbing your shin rapidly and vigorously helps with the pain. This rubbing strongly stimulates A-Beta pressure fibers again which inhibits the A-Delta and C fiber pain sensations; you feel the rubbing pressure more than the throbbing pain. You become a living, hopping example of the Pain Gate Control Theory in action.

So far, we have only addressed the ascending tract of nerves that begins at peripheral nerves and proceeds to the spinal cord and then up into the brain. There is also a descending tract from the brain down to the spinal cord. This descending tract functions primarily to decrease pain through inhibitory nerve impulses and chemicals that close pain gates. For example, oral narcotics decrease pain by causing the brain to release chemicals that send powerful inhibitory impulses to pain nerves.

Earlier, you learned that the ascending nerve fibers that cause pain sensation, travel up to the cortex and the limbic system of the brain, which are the structures responsible for thinking and feeling. As a result, thoughts and emotions can produce either excitatory or inhibitory nerve impulses that affect pain by traveling down the descending pathway. This is one way that the brain can prioritize the importance of the pain signals that it receives—usually based on the perceived threat to the body. Thus, we see the physiological basis for the fact that pain gates can either be opened or closed by thoughts and feelings.

The simplest example of the effect of thoughts and feelings on pain gates is whacking your shin on the same coffee table as mentioned before and in the same dark room, but this time, it occurs while fleeing your burning home with your newborn child in your arms. Your feelings of terror, thoughts of escape, and rush of adrenalin and other chemicals produce a massive influx of inhibitory nerve impulses. Subsequently, you may not feel much pain from your shin until you are a safe distance from your home. Your brain has said to your spinal cord and your shin, "We'll deal with that later; feet don't fail me now." Then, as the inhibition pouring down descending pathways decreases, you become acutely aware of your throbbing, aching shin; want to rub it with the arm that is not holding the baby; and wonder if your husband made it out, too.

WHAT IS NOCICEPTIVE (STIMULUS-RESPONSE) PAIN?

The spinal cord is constantly modulating painful inputs. Like individual neurons, it is bombarded with an electrical and biochemical shower of inhibitory and excitatory signals from ascending and descending nerve tracts. Painful stimuli can be produced by the external environment or internal organs, diseases, or tissue damage. These stimulus-response examples of pain transmission are referred to as nociceptive pain, and describe 99.9 percent of the human pain experience. With nociceptive pain, nerves are functioning as electrical messengers that allow an injured body part to register a formal complaint with the brain and to request assistance. Broken legs, herniated spinal discs, and touching a hot stove are all classic examples of nociceptive pain.

WHAT IS NEUROPATHIC PAIN?

The second most common category of pain is neuropathic defined as disturbance of function or pathologic change in a nerve. In other words, the nerve is not just the brain's pain messenger, but the source of the pain signal itself. Severe low back pain that radiates down a leg into the foot is neuropathic if the leg pain is caused by compression of one of the nerve roots that exit the spinal cord. In this case, even if the nerve root is decompressed by surgery so that it is no longer being injured, the patient may suffer long-term leg pain from permanent damage to the nerve root itself. Other common examples of neuropathic pain include diabetic neuropathy (diseased nerve) and neuromas (benign nerve tumor).

Neuropathic pain tends to be described as burning, electric, tingling, pins and needles, freezing, numbing, itchy, crawly, or cramping, etc. From our previous discussion, you can understand that these pain descriptors suggest that neuropathic pain is more involved with the slower, non-myelinated C fibers. The burning, tingling, pins and needles, and numbing aspect of pain is only infrequently associated with purely nociceptive pain. Therefore, if these pain descriptors accurately describe your pain, you and your doctor should suspect that some component of your pain is neuropathic in origin. Your doctor can explore various treatments that are specific to neuropathic pain, which we will discuss in later chapters.

CENTRAL AND PERIPHERAL PAIN SENSITIZATION

Since the nervous system is organized anatomically into central and peripheral systems, it makes sense that you could have central or peripheral neuropathic pain depending on the location of the affected neurons or nerve fibers. This organization allows for some unusual types of neuropathic pain. Chronic Regional Pain Syndrome or peripheral sensitization is a type of pain in which a peripheral body part becomes hypersensitive and exquisitely painful because of chronic, repeated firing of excitatory nerves with minimal input from inhibitory nerves. This can become self-perpetuating, requiring little extra outside stimulation to be maintained. Chronic Regional Pain Syndrome, Reflex Sympathetic Dystrophy, and Post Herpetic Neuralgia are examples of peripheral sensitization.

Pain from peripheral sensitization usually affects a circumscribed area like an arm, leg, or side of the face and has a burning, electric, tingling quality since it is neuropathic pain. It is usually caused by a traumatic injury that appears to have healed but leaves severe burning pain in its wake. The affected body part may become severely hypersensitive and register the slightest touch as burning pain. This is called allodynia and can be severe enough that a simple breeze or the pressure of light clothing feels like liquid fire on the skin.

Central Sensitization or Central Pain Syndrome has been called imprinted pain. Again, there is chronic over-firing of excitatory nerves with minimal input from inhibitory nerves, but at the level of the central nervous system, i.e., within the brain or spinal cord. Tragically, because the excitation is centralized, the pain may be experienced throughout the afflicted person's body or without an obvious anatomical basis.

Many amputees who have lost a limb complain of "phantom limb pain." Since the limb is missing, this cannot be a peripheral pain problem, but must be created within the brain or spinal cord. Hyper-aroused excitatory nerves continue to send pain messages in the form of electrical signals in the absence of additional input from the missing limb. This is not imaginary pain. It is no less real than stubbing your toe or breaking a bone. Fibromyalgia may be an example of an unusual type of centralized pain because it is experienced throughout the body, though usually not as a burning pain.

In a personal communication in 2005, a colleague of mine, Eola Force, R.N., used the "rutted road" analogy to describe centralized pain. Imagine a hard-baked, dirt road with deep grooves or ruts from years of use. Water will tend to flow into the ruts taking the well-worn path of least resistance. It does not matter where the water comes from; it will tend to end up in the ruts and the grooves.

Sympathetically mediated pain can be conceptualized as a combination of centralized and peripheral pain. The sympathetic nervous system is a functional system that is responsible for the body's "fight or flight" response to a threat. It includes central and peripheral nerves with most of the peripheral nerves located near the surface of the skin. Again, this pain syndrome is characterized by burning and cramping sensations along with hypersensitivity to painful stimuli, and constriction of surface blood vessels and temperature changes. However, whereas regional or peripheral pain syndromes remain in a certain limb or body part, sympathetically mediated pain can spread from limb to limb and across the torso via adjacent nerves in the sympathetic nervous system. The secondarily affected limb is called a shadow or mirror of the originally affected limb. Typically, the pain in that shadow limb is not as severe as it is in the original limb.

Peripheral, central, and sympathetically-mediated pain syndromes are examples of neuropathic pain in which some part of the body has become chronically over stimulated or excited and the normal inhibitory pain mechanisms have broken down. Why and how this happens is an issue of great controversy in the pain field. Explanations range from genetic predisposition to decreased levels of certain chemicals. However, part of the mechanism by which this happens has been demonstrated in a series of research studies related to not only neuropathic pain but also long-term nociceptive pain.

In 1994, Daniel Price et al. applied a series of painful heat impulses to subjects every three seconds and discovered that with each impulse there was a progressive increase in the total activity of neurons in the dorsal horn of the spinal cord. With each painful stimulus, more and more neurons were involved in transmitting the pain message. As you might expect, the subjects also reported escalating pain from successive heat impulses, although the intensity across impulses was maintained at a constant level.

The research by Price and his colleagues introduces the dorsal horn as an important structure in pain perception. The spinal cord consists of white and grey matter. The dorsal horn is part of the grey matter at the posterior or back end of the spinal cord. Dorsal nerve roots connect peripheral nerves to the dorsal horn of the spinal cord. Within the spinal cord, it is in the dorsal horn that pain perception is modulated by excitatory and inhibitory impulses.

The process of progressive recruitment of nerve cells in the dorsal horn that Price and his colleagues identified appears to be one way the body prioritizes the importance of a pain signal. It is likely that a repeated painful stimulus reflects a greater threat to the body than a single stimulus. However, this also demonstrates that repeated nociceptive stimuli sensitize the body to respond more strongly to future stimuli, referred to as the "wind up" phenomenon. Biochemically, an excitatory cascade overwhelms almost any inhibitory input. Moreover, inhibitory neurons in the dorsal horn of the spinal cord may become extremely inactive. This will result in dramatically increased pain perception from a painful stimulus (hyperesthesia) or, in extreme cases, pain perception from a stimulus that would not normally be painful (allodynia). This line of research also suggests that there may be increased sensitization with long-term pain that isn't nerve based, e.g., low back or neck pain.

Many patients with long-term pain believe that their pain tolerance is high and that the longer they hurt, the better they seem to tolerate their pain. In fact, the principle of sensitization and wind-up strongly suggests that biochemical pain tolerance actually decreases with the application of long-term painful stimuli. The electrical impulses and chemicals that naturally inhibit pain can become less effective over time. People who hurt for a long time are filled up with pain, and with just a little more, pain can spill over and be registered by the body as severe pain.

Mixed Pain that Combines Nociceptive and Neuropathic Elements

We have clearly distinguished between nociceptive (stimulus-response) pain and neuropathic (nerve-based) pain with the implication that painful conditions are caused by either one or the other. However, many painful conditions are a complex combination of both types of pain, referred to as mixed pain. Neck pain that radiates into your arms following injury probably has both nociceptive and neuropathic elements. The same is true of back pain that radiates down your leg. A mix of nociceptive and neuropathic elements often causes headaches. Mixed pain certainly complicates the process of diagnosis and treatment.

The average physician is much more familiar with short-term, nociceptive pain conditions than neuropathic pain or long-term nociceptive pain. The average patient is completely unfamiliar with the other types of pain that are long-term or neuropathic in origin. These other pain conditions do not look like typical, short-term nociceptive pain. Often, the pain is reported to be more severe than objective medical testing and physical examination would seem to warrant. Thus, patients with neuropathic or long-term nociceptive pain may often be treated with disbelief or suspicion by the doctors who initially treat their condition. The doctors may perceive them as "psych" patients who are either somaticizing their pain or grossly exaggerating their pain severity. Neither of these perceptions is accurate but they can severely compromise quality of care and cause unnecessary patient suffering.

This chapter provided the physiological underpinnings of several critical facts about pain and its treatment. First, how much pain you have is determined not just by the excitatory signals of tissue injury but also by how powerful the inhibitory signals are. Second, nerves can simply carry the pain message or be the source of the pain message. Third, long-term pain can sensitize the body to painful stimuli. Fourth, many pain conditions are a mix of tissue injury and nerve-based pain.

My understanding of various types of pain can improve my medical care

Insight—I understand the difference between nociceptive and neuropathic pain.
Commitment—I will evaluate my own pain condition from this new perspective.
Action—I will discuss this new information with my doctor and clarify her understanding of my type of pain and how that should affect my treatment.
Now—I will document my evaluation and my questions for the doctor in my TAAP journal.

3

The Differences between Acute and Chronic Pain

For thousands of years, long-term pain was a "dirty little secret" that was ignored by society in general and doctors specifically. In the 1950s and 60s, medical researchers began looking at long-term pain and how best to treat it. Fifty years' worth of research and clinical experience later, we know a lot more about long-term pain and understand that there are differences in how it should be treated, compared with short-term pain. Unfortunately, the majority of physicians still do not have this information and the vast majority of medical patients, long-term pain sufferers, and their families are uninformed as well.

Short-term pain tends to be nociceptive, i.e., the injury tends to heal and the pain disappears. Neuropathic pain, especially sympathetically mediated pain and both peripheral and central pain syndromes are self-perpetuating, often in the face of maximal healing, so the pain is much more likely to continue for a long time. In particular, it is often impossible to eliminate centralized and sympathetically mediated pain that has spread to other body areas. A reasonable treatment goal for long-term pain, even ongoing nociceptive pain, is more likely to be pain reduction rather than pain elimination.

As your treatment proceeds through the levels of the W.H.O. ladder, you most likely will have experienced pain for a long period of time. The longer you have suffered pain, the more risk and side effects you may be willing to accept in exchange for pain relief. Additionally, the further you proceed up the W.H.O. ladder, the more likely it is that healthy treatment goals have changed from complete pain elimination to significant pain relief. For example, you probably had pain for a long time before you were placed on really strong, continuous release narcotics, or were referred to a pain psychologist. When you are referred for a spinal cord stimulator or implantable pump, your doctor has long since concluded

24

that some element of your pain is permanent, or at least will continue into the near future.

WHAT IS ACUTE PAIN?

Short-term pain is almost always nociceptive and is also called acute pain stemming from the Latin word, meaning needle, or sharp. You have seen that it can be caused by injury such as a sprained ankle or by illness such as a sinus infection, pneumonia, kidney stone, or gastric ulcer. It can be anything from a mild annoyance to an agony with dripping fangs.

Most importantly, acute pain serves as a warning signal to your body that you are being injured and that you need to take steps to protect yourself. It is a warning signal that has powerful survival value. If you set your hand on a hot stove, the searing pain tells you that your hand is being injured and that you need to remove it. This communication from hand to brain and back down to hand happens in milliseconds, and does not require conscious thought on your part. Your body reacts by reflex and you pull your hand away from the heat.

In this context, acute, nociceptive pain is generally positive, healthy, and adaptive. It is good and life affirming. It has and will continue to save your life. It communicates something important to you—that you need to take action. The chest pain you feel from pneumonia or a blocked heart vessel will drive you into the doctor's office for the treatment that can make the difference between life and death. So, acute pain is your friend. Hooray for acute pain.

What is the Relationship between Acute Pain and Healing?

Thank goodness, acute pain goes away. It always goes away. Well, almost always. If we were to graph what acute pain looks like, it would be described as shown in Figure 1. The amount of pain is represented by the up and down or vertical (Y) axis with length of time indicated by the side-to-side or horizontal (X) axis.

Figure 1: Acute Pain over Time

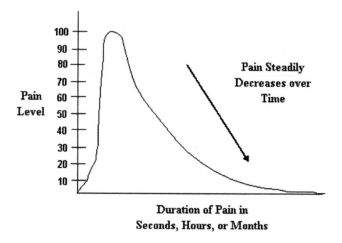

Duration of Pain in
Seconds, Hours, or Months

In this graph, acute pain is seen as peaking or spiking very quickly after injury and then steadily decreasing over time until it goes away. The pain of a stubbed toe comes on almost instantaneously, peaks for a few seconds, and then drops quickly in seconds or minutes, though it can take hours or days to disappear completely. Therefore, acute pain is rather predictable. As time passes, the pain is almost always less than it was before. The fact that it steadily gets better is called tonic, not like gin and tonic, but meaning steady and predictable. Acute pain predictably and invariably gets better because the body is healing from the injury, and with healing, comes improved function and decreased pain.

Figure 2 shows the common sense relationship between function and pain in an individual with acute pain. Function is on the vertical (Y) axis and pain is on the horizontal (X) axis.

Figure 2: Relationship between Pain Level and Functional Ability

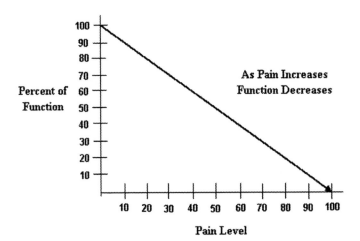

The more pain a person has, the less she can function. The less pain a person has, the more she can function. In this context, pain limits a person's ability to function and is partly independent of tissue damage. With a badly sprained ankle, damage to tendons or ligaments certainly affects the ability to bear weight or walk. Nevertheless, the increased pain experienced from bearing weight or walking is also a limiting factor.

With pain from almost any source, function improves and pain decreases because of healing until the body heals completely and the pain goes away. At this point, I should note that all the standard medical treatments for acute pain assume that acute pain is usually nociceptive and stems from tissue damage that is naturally healing. Thus, the role of medical treatment with acute pain is to facilitate natural healing or control the pain until the healing process finishes, complete function has been restored, and pain has ended.

What Is the Relationship Between Acute Pain and Tissue Damage?

The fact that acute pain steadily decreases over time and with healing means that there is a strong correlation between the amount of tissue damage and the amount of pain within individual people. A lot of tissue damage hurts intensely; a little tissue damage (from either a small injury or partial healing) mostly just hurts a little. But, this is also true for different people with pain. We describe this relationship in Figure 3 where the X-axis represents the amount of tissue damage and the amount of pain is determined by the Y-axis. We document 100 patients on this graph where each point represents the intersection of a particular patient's pain level and tissue damage. Notice that the graph line goes from the bottom left to the top right. This means that as tissue damage increases, so does the pain level. Conversely, as tissue damage decreases across the group, so does the pain.

Figure 3: Relationship between Acute Pain Level and Amount of Tissue Damage

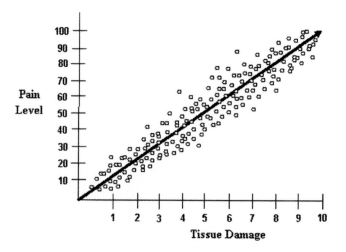

In Figure 3, notice also how closely grouped or clustered the dots are. For the vast majority of people with acute pain, the intersection of pain level and tissue damage is very close to the centerline that runs through all of them. This means that there is a very strong correlation between the amount of tissue damage and the amount of pain. In other words, when you have acute pain, how much pain you feel is almost entirely dependent upon how badly you hurt yourself; your pain level is not much affected by other factors. Some researchers have noted that about 80 percent of the pain you feel with acute injury is directly caused by the amount of injury. Duh! This is just good, common sense.

On the other hand, we must keep in mind that 20 percent of the pain you feel with acute injury is caused by factors other than how badly you got hurt. Like what? Well, genetics and basic pain tolerance play a role. There are individual differences in how effectively the dorsal horn (posterior spinal cord) regulates pain. Emotional and situational variables can also affect pain perception via the descending pain tract from the cortex and limbic structures of the brain down the dorsal horn. All these factors affect the flux of excitatory and inhibitory impulses received by the neurons in the dorsal horn and the opening and closing of pain gates.

You certainly have had thousands of experiences with acute pain episodes that required anywhere from seconds to months to go away. The length of time depends on how long it takes the body to heal enough to be pain free following an injury. We cannot predict how long acute pain will last, but we do know that the body does not continue to heal itself forever. At some point, the healing ends, and tragically enough, sometimes this happens with a degree of long-term damage and subsequent pain. This may occur because of continuing nociceptive impulses or because of the development of chronic neuropathic pain. How long tissue damage will continue to heal varies depending mostly on the type and location of the injury.

How Long Does It Take Acute Tissue Damage to Heal?

Statistically speaking, especially for nerve, muscle, joint, tendon, or bone injury, the vast majority of healing naturally occurs within three to six months. With classic injury, like a strained low back or sore neck that is severe enough to require a visit to the doctor, about 90-95 percent of patients are fully recovered and pain free within six months. An additional 4-8 percent of patients require between about six and twelve months to become pain free. About 1 percent of patients become pain free after a year, and about 1 percent are never completely pain free. This last 1 percent includes the patients who continue to experience long-term nociceptive pain, or who have developed chronic neuropathic pain, including peripheral or central pain syndrome, or sympathetically mediated pain.

Generally, the body naturally heals about as much as it ever will within a 0-12 month window. If you have experienced pain for a year or longer, the likelihood of complete, pain-free recovery is small and becoming smaller with the passage of time. If you've had pain for years, the odds of a full and pain-free recovery are almost nonexistent. Let's just sit with that for a bit before we proceed. I will wait.

(Ouch. This sucks. He has no bedside manner. What a miserable way to encourage me. I want to read one of the books that promises "Freedom from Pain Effortlessly in 30 Days or Less!")

Now hold on a minute. First, the authors who write such books are liars—stealing your money while preying on your desperation. Second, we said "naturally healing" and "complete recovery." You and your doctors can do many things to help your body "un-naturally" heal even more, although that is a weird way to describe it. In terms of recovery and pain relief, would you settle for 50 percent pain relief, 70 percent, or 90 percent? Actually, you can't exactly settle for it. You have to work very hard for it and your doctors probably can't give it to you. But, I'm getting ahead of myself.

RATING YOUR PAIN

Let's try another exercise. In the space below, I would like you to rate the severity of your pain right this moment on a scale of 0-100, where 0 is absolutely pain free everywhere and 100 is the worst pain you have ever experienced in your entire life.

Now on that same scale of 0-100, I would like you to write down the two numbers that your pain fluctuates between in a typical day. What is the best and worst it gets more days than not, during regular waking hours? Finally, I would like you to write down your average level of pain on the 0-100 scale over the past thirty days.

My immediate pain as I sit here is about a _____ on a scale of 0-100. On a typical day, my pain varies between about a low of _____/100 and a high of _____/100. Over the past thirty days, my waking pain has averaged about a _____ on a scale of 0-100.

WHAT IS CHRONIC PAIN?

Pain that lingers after six to twelve months is called chronic pain—not acute pain that refuses to go away. It looks, smells, and tastes different, because it **is** different.

Remember, acute pain is a warning signal that communicates valuable information to the brain about the body. We refer to acute pain as tonic because it is steadily getting better as the body heals. With chronic pain, the body does not heal naturally and steadily anymore. It has done about as much healing as it can. So, chronic pain does not steadily do anything.

If chronic pain were just acute pain that didn't go away, it might look like the example in Figure 4. This shows one person's acute pain condition, i.e., a herniated lumbar disc that does not go away and remains steadily the same forever. However, if you have chronic pain, you know that Figure 4 is nonsense. That is not what your pain does. It varies, probably a lot, based on numerous factors, including how you slept the night before, how active you are, and what the weather is like outside.

Figure 4: Hypothesized Relationship between Chronic Pain Level and Time

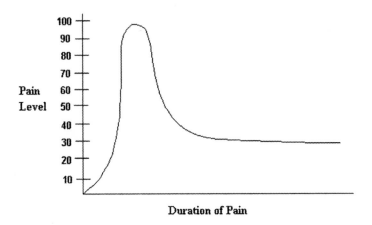

Chronic pain actually looks like Figure 5, where we have an acute pain that continues and begins to vary, to wax and wane, like the tides or phases of the moon. You can have bad hours, days, weeks, or seasons. Some people have a unipolar pain pattern with a single pain peak during a typical day. They may hurt worse in the morning with decreased pain throughout the day. Some people hurt more as a day progresses, especially with activity. Some people hurt more in the morning, feel better about mid day, and hurt more again in the evening (the truly cursed). This latter pattern is called a bipolar pain pattern because it has two peaks of more severe pain. Regardless of the pain pattern, chronic pain is referred to as phasic because it varies like the tides or a sine wave in trigonometry.

This point cannot be emphasized enough. Chronic pain varies. It always varies, and it usually varies a lot. When I interview patients for the first time, I ask them, "How much does your pain vary or fluctuate? On a scale of 1-100, if 100 is the most severe pain you've ever had, what's the least your pain gets and what's the most it gets on a typical day, more days than not?" The most common response is a range between 40 and 80, a difference of 40. Since I know that pain varies a lot, I am looking for a difference of at least 30. I want to determine if my patients know that their pain varies considerably over a day, a week, or a month.

Look at the two numbers that you wrote that reflect how much your pain varies during a typical day. Subtract the low number from the high number and see how much variation you endorsed. If you stated that your pain varies less than 30, you are probably wrong. In a typical day, from the time you get up in the morning to the time you go to bed at night, your pain will vary 30 or more. Recognizing this daily variation in pain level is vital to effective pain treatment and management.

Figure 5: Actual Relationship between Chronic Pain and Time

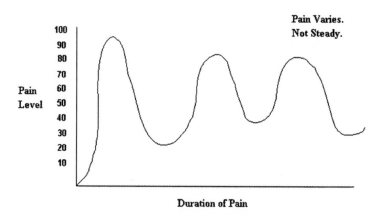

If you do not notice that your pain varies, you will be unable to evaluate the effectiveness of any treatment. Thus, as long as you have any pain, you will be unable to feel hopeful or encouraged about small changes in pain relief. If you stated that your pain is always a 70, 80, or 90/100 or that it only varies ten or twenty points, you are already in deep trouble. In this event, it is absolutely vital that you frequently pay attention to your pain over the next few weeks so you can better appreciate the changes in your pain levels. In my experience, the greater the range of pain variation of which you are aware, the more control you will eventually be able to exert over your pain.

What Is the Relationship Between Chronic Pain and Tissue Damage?

We noted that in a group of people with acute pain, there was a strong relationship between the amount of tissue damage and the amount of pain. In Figure 3, we saw that people with increased tissue damage almost inevitably had greater pain with very little variation or effect from other factors (20 percent or less).

However, we can see in Figure 6 that the relationship between chronic tissue damage and pain looks different. Patient scores are much less clustered around the centerline and much more spread out. Generally, it still appears that the more tissue damage our group has, the more pain they have. But, we have some other people with severe damage and a little pain, and quite a few more people with a little damage and a lot more pain.

Figure 6: Relationship between Chronic Pain Level and Amount of Tissue Damage

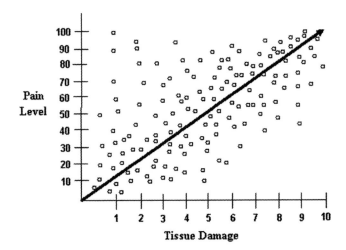

With chronic pain, the relationship between the amount of tissue damage and the amount of pain is much weaker. Researchers have concluded that between 30 percent and 70 percent of chronic pain is due to factors other than the original tissue damage. This means that with chronic pain, factors other than the original injury or tissue damage play a much more dominant role in how much pain you have. These factors may include the development of neuropathic types of pain or the sensitization and "wind-up" we discussed in the last chapter. More commonly, these factors may be caused by your body's adjustment to your pain. The following example may be helpful.

John was a 48-year-old construction worker who injured his low back and had undergone several spine surgeries. A right-sided nerve root exiting his spine had been crushed causing radiculopathy, a neuropathic pain in his right leg. For years, he had favored his right leg when he stood or walked because putting weight on his right leg caused him much more pain. He habitually bore most of his weight on his left leg. With almost any activity, even sitting, he tended to use his left leg and left side low back muscles more than his right due to his right side pain.

Over time, John's right leg and right side low back became weaker and began to atrophy. His left leg and left side low back developed overuse syndrome since they were compensating for the right side. Basic posture and body mechanics became increasingly distorted as his right leg became shorter from atrophy and pelvic shifting. Inevitably, he ended up with increased back pain due to his distorted posture. He also developed pain in his left hip and left knee due to overcompensation for the right side. All of this happened in the absence of any increased tissue damage to the disc or spine that was left over from his last surgery. This complication from chronic pain simply does not occur with a brief, acute pain condition. Nevertheless, such a complication can lead to severely increasing chronic pain with no additional damage to the original injured tissue.

WHAT ARE THE DIFFERENCES BETWEEN ACUTE AND CHRONIC PAIN?

We learned in an earlier chapter that acute, nociceptive pain is the result of three sets of nerve fibers that are progressively slower: A-Beta, A-Delta, and C fibers. The A-Beta fibers follow the neospinothalamic path in the brain, which extends into the thalamus and cortex. The A-Delta and C fibers follow the paleospinothalamic pathway that extends into the hypothalamus and limbic structures of the brain.

Chronic pain uses almost exclusively the A-Delta and C fibers along the paleospinothalamic path. Moreover, chronic pain tends to "light up" the C fibers much more than the A-Delta fibers, which explains the deep aching, throbbing, cramping, or burning sensations of classic chronic pain. Thus, at a fundamental anatomic and biochemical level, acute and chronic pain do different things in different places in the body.

The important lesson to be learned from the above discussion is that acute and chronic pain are not the same thing. Chronic pain is not simply acute pain that does not go away. Acute pain is a warning signal; chronic pain is not. Acute pain communicates something necessary, adaptive, and even life affirming. Chronic pain does not. Acute pain is steady or tonic, while chronic pain is variable or phasic.

With acute pain, there is a strong relationship between tissue damage and pain—not so with chronic pain. Acute pain almost always gets better. Chronic pain often gets worse. Acute and chronic pains tend to follow different paths in the brain. Chronic pain is much more likely than acute pain to produce increased excitatory impulses at the dorsal horn with decreased inhibitory impulses. The pain gates are more likely to stay wide open.

If short-and long-term pain were not the same thing, then why would the treatments for acute pain make chronic pain go away? The answer is that they do not. The treatments for acute pain can be helpful for chronic pain, but they are insufficient at best and occasionally destructive at worst. I see pain patients every day who are worse off because of the well-intended treatments they have received. In the next chapter, we turn our attention to medical treatments that were developed for acute pain, but are also used for chronic pain.

I can use my understanding of chronic pain to establish realistic goals

Insight—I understand the difference between acute and chronic pain and that my pain is chronic pain.

Commitment—I will hope for a pain cure in the future, but will focus my efforts on decreasing my pain and improving my ability to function.

Action—For the next few weeks, I will pay close attention to my daily pain pattern.

Now—I will document my pain pattern and other information in my TAAP journal.

4

Medical Treatments for Acute Pain

If you have wrestled with physical pain for more than a year, you have probably received a half dozen or so of the treatments listed on the W.H.O. ladder, and been less than satisfied with some or all of them. As each of them failed, you may have felt more and more discouraged, as if confronting an enemy for the first time that you could not understand or conquer. Your doctors and therapists, perhaps even your own family, may have given you the look that says, "What's wrong with you? Don't you want to get better?" If you do not have pain in your neck, shoulders, or arms, pat yourself on the back for not smacking these people. We will discuss them again later.

WHAT ARE THE MAJOR SOURCES OF PAIN?

Treatments for both nociceptive and neuropathic pain can be directed toward either minimizing or eliminating the underlying pain source or simply masking the pain itself. With neuropathic pain, we know that the nerves themselves are the source of the pain, but there are several possible sources of nociceptive pain. The most important and common source of pain is inflammation.

Inflammatory Pain

My colleague, Vernon Williams, M.D., is the Director of the Pain Program at the Kerlan Jobe Orthopedic Clinic in Los Angeles. In a personal communication in 2004, he stated, "With most injury, inflammation is usually the trigger for initiating pain signals and sensitizing nerves. We now have blood tests available that can indicate the level of global inflammation present in a person's body. Controlling inflammation is often the key to controlling pain."

When you injure a part of your body, a signal is sent from the affected body part to the brain via the ascending tract. The brain causes the release of chemicals around and toward the site of injury, which includes dilation of blood vessels in the affected area and leakage of plasma and white blood cells into the surrounding tissues. Inflammation is largely an immune system response meant to destroy foreign bodies that also uses swelling as a protective mechanism to minimize risk of additional injury.

For instance, when a joint is injured, part of the healing process requires that the joint be immobilized. Swelling minimizes how much the joint can move around. Unfortunately, inflammation and associated swelling also produce pain. We know that it can be helpful to minimize swelling from a sprained ankle and that we should protect the ankle from further injury through the RICE strategy of Rest, Ice, Compression, and Elevation. The protective mechanism of swelling actually does more harm than good if we know enough to protect the injured site through our behavior. With chronic pain, it is important to continue to use the injured body part and ongoing inflammation can impede such use.

Muscle-Based Pain

Another source of pain is muscle tissue. A muscle pull, strain, or tear can cause pain, independent of inflammation. This is especially true when the muscle does not heal quickly and the acute inflammatory process ends before the muscle is completely healed.

There are two types of muscle. Striated muscle is working muscle in the outer regions of the body that allows you to voluntarily move, lift, bend, etc. Smooth muscle is inside the body and helps involuntary processes like undulating peristalsis, which propels food through the stomach and the intestines. It is usually the striated muscle that is injured and causing pain.

Covering every inch of striated muscle is the fascia, a flexible, fibrous coating that protects the muscle. Often, what is diagnosed as muscle strain is actually a stretching or tearing of the fascia. This is true with many neck injuries caused by violent motion of the head, referred to as whiplash. Myofascial pain is a generic term referring to pain in the muscle or fascia.

Often, muscle pain is reflected in trigger points which David Alvarez and Pamela Rockwell (2002) refer to as discrete, focal, hyper-irritable spots located in a tight band in the middle of skeletal muscle. These are painful when compressed. Such compression also causes referred pain in the surrounding area and a twitchy response when the band is snapped by a perpendicular pressure. The presence of trigger points is indicative of myofascial pain.

Trigger points are distinguished from tender points, which are also painful to compression. However, tender points do not produce referred pain and occur at insertion points in the muscle, not in tight bands in the middle of the muscle. Tender points almost always occur in multiple areas and their presence is a necessary criteria for diagnosis of Fibromyalgia.

Connective Tissue Pain

The third major source of pain is injury to connective tissue such as tendons or ligaments. Tendons connect muscle to bone. Ligaments connect two structures, usually one bone to another, to help create a joint. Stretching or tearing these connectors can cause pain. In the spine, this can be referred to as ligamental derangement. Tendons and ligaments usually require a long time to heal, and they often do not heal completely. A severely sprained ankle that badly strains tendons may be more vulnerable to another sprain for years, or even forever.

Skeletal Pain

Another potential source of pain is injury to skeletal (bone) or bony substances. A fractured arm or spinal vertebrae can cause excruciating pain and require immediate treatment. You might injure your tailbone (coccyx), or have a herniated vertebral disc. If the injury heals fully, you may end up pain free, but the site of injury will not recover to its original pre-injury condition.

Vascular and Miscellaneous Pain

Another potential trigger for pain lies in the vascular system. Damage to blood vessels, especially constriction or explosive expansion (dilation) can cause pain. Examples of this type of pain include chest pain caused by constricted or blocked heart arteries, and migraine headaches associated with constriction and then explosive dilation of blood vessels in the brain. This type of pain is more likely to be episodic, i.e., to come and go.

There are miscellaneous sources of pain including organ damage such as might be found from stomach ulcers or kidney stones. Scar tissue can also cause pain mainly by restricting normal movement or function of other body parts. An example is scar tissue in the spine following surgery, sometimes loosely referred to as arachnoiditis.

Neuropathic Pain

Of course, the final source of pain is in the nerves themselves, i.e., neuropathic pain. You know that all pain is perceived and regulated through nerve cells in the central and peripheral nervous systems that allow the brain and the injured body part to communicate. However, when the nerves themselves are injured, the pain is often described as burning, searing, tingling, or cramping. It may be associated with numbness or tingling as well. Nerve-based pain is not necessarily worse than other types of pain, but nerve injury can cause pain in areas far removed from the site of injury. For instance, I mentioned that damage to a nerve root that exits the lumbar spine could cause pain all the way down a leg and into the toes.

Pain can affect multiple types of tissue. Medical treatment of both acute and chronic pain aims to heal or reduce the influence of all these pain triggers.

THE FIVE MAJOR TREATMENTS FOR ACUTE PAIN

We can now turn our attention to the five major categories of medical treatment that are more effective for acutely painful conditions:

1. Surgery

2. Physical Therapy

3. Injections for Pain

4. Narcotic Medications

5. Non-narcotic Medications

These categories are presented from a slightly different perspective than the W.H.O. ladder in terms of their potential power to eliminate pain or heal injury.

Surgery

Surgery is the most powerful and most invasive option for many types of pain relief. Surgery holds the promise of cure for many kinds of pain, perhaps the best examples being appendicitis, inguinal hernia, gallbladder attacks, and severe coronary artery disease. In the field of medicine, the surgeon is the closest physician to the Divine Creator. With their feet on the ground, surgeons can reach their magnificent hands to the heavens, tilt their heads back, and roar at the gods, "You don't get this one; not for awhile yet." And by the way, your pain is gone.

Surgeons do not directly treat pain. They cut, eliminate, add, or reshape living tissue. With very few exceptions, surgeons do not return the human body back to its natural healthy state. Rather, they try to craft living tissue in a way that will be as close as possible to natural, fully functioning tissue. The vast majority of surgery has as its principal goal to improve function, save lives, or increase longevity. Pain relief is usually a highly desirable or assumed side effect of surgery. Even when pain relief is the principal goal, it is a desired effect of crafting living tissue. Ultimately, surgery treats tissue, not pain.

A surgeon once told me, "If you perform surgery only for pain, that's exactly what you'll get." This statement reflects the fact that surgery for the sole purpose of pain relief has a very uncertain outcome. The longer you have suffered from pain, the less likely it is that surgery will dramatically relieve or eliminate your pain. Remember, the longer you have experienced pain, the more likely it is that factors other than tissue damage are major contributors or triggers for your pain. Because surgery can only treat tissue, the less your pain is tissue based, the less likely it is that surgery will help you. In the extreme case, if 70 percent of your pain is not due to tissue damage, surgery may be able to help with at most 30 percent of your problem, and that is with a nearly perfect outcome.

The statistics with low back surgeries are illustrative. Some researchers have suggested that about 90 percent of first spinal surgeries bring complete pain relief and recovery of function. About 50 percent of second spinal surgeries produce complete relief and full function. Less than 10 percent of third spinal surgeries result in complete freedom from pain. By the time you are a candidate for your third spinal surgery, you have endured two post surgical regimens and have probably had pain for at least two to four years. By that time, there are most likely multiple physical sources or triggers for your pain. You probably have some combination of inflammatory, muscle, tendon or ligament, joint, and nerve-based pain with multiple other pain triggers. Additionally, some of the tissue damage in your spine may be permanent and irreversible.

Pain doctors call this constellation of pain triggers "multifactoral." Most surgeons probably do not believe that you will be pain free or "as good as new" after a third spinal surgery, hernia repair, or abdominal surgery for scar tissue, but they may believe that you will have less pain and be more functional, as is true of most patients. However, many patients will undergo that third spinal surgery believing that anything less than complete pain relief is a failure. In this situation, the goals of the patient and the surgeon do not match, and the patient is likely to be unhappy with the outcome.

I evaluated a patient in his late '50s who had undergone twenty-six spinal surgeries, mostly for pain relief. He was referred by his surgeon for psychological screening prior to his twenty-seventh surgery. When we discussed his treatment goals, he made it clear that he expected complete pain relief and said that if he didn't get it, he would find another surgeon who would perform his twenty-eighth surgery. Since he had a better chance of giving birth to twins than being pain free, I did not clear him psychologically for surgery, and his very wise referring surgeon did not operate. I suspect the patient later found a surgeon who did.

The bottom line is that a significant percentage of patients with acute pain who undergo surgery continue to have pain. An even greater percentage of patients with chronic pain continue to have pain after surgery. This does not mean that your surgeon made a mistake or that anyone committed malpractice. Assuming that you are a good person, it just means that bad things happen to good people, or that your expectations for surgery were too high.

I have worked with thousands of patients who were dissatisfied with a surgical outcome. In a large percentage of those cases, the surgeon was perfectly content with the outcome of the tissue crafting, i.e., the hernia was fully repaired or the spinal fusion was solid and stable. In many cases, if the patient had known that successful tissue crafting could leave significant residual pain, the patient might not have proceeded with the surgery. The patient may know there is a chance of residual pain but probably assumes that pain will continue only if the tissue crafting is unsuccessful or poorly done.

The quality of communication between surgeons and patients is often poor, and at least as much the fault of patients as it is surgeons. Many of my patients have been told by their surgeon, "There's an 80 percent chance of a successful surgery," without any idea how the surgeon defines success. His idea of performing "typical" activities may not include mountain biking or beach volleyball. When the surgeon says, "You'll be back to work in six months," patients often assume that returning to work means being fully recovered. It doesn't. We will discuss this more in later chapters.

Physical Therapy

Many patients who have acute or chronic pain will be referred for a course of physical, occupational, or water therapy. Physical therapy is a branch of rehabilitative health that uses special equipment and/or exercises to help patients regain physical ability. The primary measuring stick and goals for physical therapy are increased strength, range of motion, and physical endurance. This means moving more weight across a greater range of movement, for a longer period. This is a very powerful treatment modality for injury and dysfunction.

Traditionally, physical therapists were highly competent medical professionals who completed a rigorous four to five-year college program of education and clinical training. More recently, physical therapists have Master's or Doctoral degrees reflecting even greater education and training.

You now know that the goals of physical therapy are increased strength, range of motion, and endurance. In the pain classes I teach, I always ask my patients what they believe to be the goal of physical therapy. Inevitably, they mention pain relief, usually as the first goal. Unfortunately, this is not true. Why the misunderstanding? Most pain patients go to physical therapy because they hurt and they want to hurt less. They assume the therapist has the same goal.

Physical therapy is a treatment developed mainly for acute injury or disease, to help a naturally healing body heal faster and reach healthy function. Sometimes people are referred to physical therapy for weakness, which is not necessarily associated with pain or formal injury. Most often, however, people are referred after an injury or surgery when they do have pain and want to have less.

Remember from Figure 1 that in a naturally healing body, pain is decreasing because of healing which takes place over <u>time</u>. Decreased pain is an inevitable consequence of healing, improved function, and the passage of time. Figure 2 indicated that with acute pain, decreasing pain is associated with improving function, especially when pain is a limiting factor. Thus, with the vast majority of physical therapy patients, pain relief is an inevitable product or side effect of increased function in a healing body as measured by strength, range of motion, and endurance over time.

However, the tissue damage that causes chronic pain is no longer naturally healing, so chronic pain is not steadily getting better with the simple passage of time. In Figure 3, we noted a very strong relationship between the amount of acute pain and the amount of tissue damage. This is also reflected in the inverse relationship between pain and function. Increasing pain decreases function and decreasing pain increases function.

In Figure 6, however, we saw that the relationship between chronic pain and tissue damage was weaker. There are more people with high tissue damage and low pain, but even more people with relatively little tissue damage and worse pain. This means that with chronic pain, the inverse relationship between pain and function also gets weaker.

With chronic pain, increasing pain usually causes decreasing function, but not always and not as consistently. Some long-term pain sufferers have only mild to moderate baseline pain that they have learned is made much worse by activity, so they severely limit their activity to maintain relatively mild levels of pain, i.e., they have relatively low pain with very low functioning. Other patients may have rather severe pain all the time and do not notice much of an increase in pain with activity, so they can be relatively active in spite of their rather severe pain, i.e., they have high pain with relatively high functioning.

When physical therapy is provided to patients with chronic pain patterns, the outcome is utterly uncertain. In my practice, about 75 percent of patients say that physical therapy increased their pain even though it may have dramatically improved their function. This is another example of a pain pattern with increasing pain in spite of increasing function. This happens because much of the pain is residual from permanent damage or multifactoral in origin, and physical therapy simply cannot address all these pain issues—no single treatment can. With chronic pain, most patients will describe physical therapy as a failure even if it improves function as long as it increases or does not decrease physical pain. This is a misperception since physical therapy was never intended as a treatment primarily for the purpose of pain reduction. We see patient dissatisfaction when the goals of the patient and the medical provider are different.

The process of physical therapy is further complicated by the realities of insurance authorizations and utilization reviews. To justify continued physical therapy treatments to insurance companies, physical therapists need to demonstrate improvements in strength, flexibility, and endurance almost every week. If your pain is of several years' duration, it may take several years of slowly graduated exercise to make significant gains. Physical therapists cannot take this long. They are allowed a limited number of treatment sessions and time, usually about twelve to twenty-four sessions over a two to four month period. This is probably faster than your body can tolerate making dramatic gains.

For many people with chronic pain, physical therapy becomes something they endure to be good, compliant patients for as long as it is prescribed. When it blessedly ends, they collapse in a chair for a few weeks and try to get back to the baseline level of pain they had before it started, whereupon they lose any gains in function achieved through therapy. This is a treatment disaster and really no one's fault. It simply reflects the fact that traditional physical therapy was developed for acute, naturally healing medical conditions, not chronic pain.

However, you should know that some physical therapists have learned how to treat patients with chronic pain. This means that they are committed to types and levels of exercise that do not increase pain. Their work is educational as much as treatment oriented with some emphasis on what you can continue to do after physical therapy has ended. These are the physical therapists with whom you want to work. In a 2005 communication, my colleague Sandy Cameron, M.P.T., noted that, "I want my patients with chronic pain to learn that exercise doesn't have to hurt, that they can become longer and stronger without hurting worse. Then they will continue to exercise on their own."

Injections for Pain

Many patients with acute pain will receive injections of various kinds. Cortisone or steroid injections can reduce or eliminate inflammatory pain. Epidural injections are steroid injections into the epidural space of the spine. Muscle-based pain from trigger or tender points may be treated with local injections using an anesthetic agent, like Lidocaine or Marcaine (Bupivicaine). If patients obtain significant benefit from these anesthetic injections, they may be candidates for Botox injections, which use a low dose of the botulism bacteria to paralyze the affected muscles for several months and provide even longer-term pain relief.

Certain types of joint pain may benefit from joint injections using steroids or some of the newer medications. Synvisc is a viscous fluid made from a substance found in normal joints that can help lubricate and provide pain relief if injected into the knee. Some doctors are injecting stem cells into aching joints to promote healing and provide pain relief. If the facet joints of the spine are a pain trigger, facet injections may be helpful. If facet injections are pain relieving, the doctor may consider radio frequency ablation (destruction) of the facet nerve. If an element of your pain is neuropathic, selective nerve root blocks, stellate ganglion blocks, or other types of injections may help to reduce or eliminate pain.

As is true of most treatments, the longer you have hurt, the less likely it is that injections of any type will provide permanent, complete pain relief. Injections are still important to consider with chronic pain if they can provide even a little permanent relief or several months of significant partial relief. If even temporary pain relief is achieved, physical therapy or other exercise may be easier and yield additional long-term benefits.

Narcotic Medications

The fourth and fifth treatments for acute pain are medications that are not inject-able, mainly oral medication. These drugs provide analgesia (pain relief) by either treating the underlying pain trigger or by simply masking the pain caused by the pain trigger. There are many different categories of analgesics. For our purposes, we begin by differentiating between narcotics and non-narcotics.

Narcotics never really treat the underlying pain trigger, but mask pain at the level of the dorsal horn of the spinal cord. Narcotics (synthetic opioids) always require a prescription. The body produces natural opioids, like endorphins and enkephalins. These chemicals function by blocking pain receptors and inhibiting the pain messages from reaching the brain. They close pain gates. Narcotics are manufactured chemicals that also block pain receptors from sending pain mes-sages to the brain, hence, the term synthetic opioid.

Generally, there are three classes of prescription opioid medications: the sim-ple codeine-based medications, the Oxycodone branch, and the Hydrocodone branch. Any opioid whose name ends in *cet* contains ace*t*aminophen in addition to the base opioid. In my patient population, the hierarchy of common oral opi-oid medications from weakest to strongest is:

- Darvon, Darvocet (Propoxyphene)

- Tylenol with Codeine; #3, #4

- Ultram, Ultracet (Tramadol—highly atypical narcotic)

- Lortab, Lorcet (Hydrocodone)

- Vicodin (Hydrocodone with Tylenol), Vicoprofen (Hydrocodone with Ibu-profen)

- Norco (Hydrocodone branch)

- Percodan, Percocet (Oxycodone)

- OxyContin (continuous release Oxycodone),

- Oxy IR (instant release Oxycodone)

- MS Contin, Kadian, Avinza (continuous release morphine sulfate) (Hydro-codone)

- MSIR (instant release morphine sulfate) (Hydrocodone)

- Methadone (Hydrocodone)

- Dilaudid (Hydrocodone)

Another strong opioid is Fentanyl, though not taken in pill form. Fentanyl can be taken in lollipop form and absorbed through the gums as Actiq, or as a patch worn on the skin for two to three days called Duragesic. With acute pain, these narcotics are used when the patient cannot take oral narcotics for some reason, such as the inability to swallow or when experiencing gastrointestinal side effects.

Narcotics are especially effective for nociceptive (stimulus-response) types of pain, much less so for neuropathic (nerve-based) pain. Any narcotic taken daily for a month or longer almost inevitably produces physical dependence and tolerance. This is not the same as addiction, which we will discuss later.

Non-narcotic Pain Medications

The two general types of non-narcotic medications are those that are curative and those that are simply analgesic, or pain relieving. Antibiotics are an example of curative medication. If you have pain caused solely by an infection, oral antibiotics like Vancomycin, Zithromax (azithromycin), etc., can eliminate the infection and cure the pain. A simple, one-time tension headache may be essentially "cured" by a variety of headache medications from aspirin to Tylenol.

ANTI-INFLAMMATORIES

Non-narcotic, analgesic medications can be divided into anti-inflammatories, used primarily for pain caused by inflammation, and non-anti-inflammatories. Anti-inflammatories include both steroidal and non-steroidal anti-inflammatories (NSAIDs). The most common oral steroid for inflammatory pain is the Medrol Dose Pack, which is taken over a period of five days. Prescription non-steroidal anti-inflammatories include the new Cox-2 inhibitor Celebrex (Celecoxib) as well as older medications like Feldene (Piroxicam), Clinoril (Sulidac), Dolobid (Diflunisal), Voltaren (Diclofenac), and Mobic (Meloxicam). Most research has demonstrated the efficacy of the Cox-2 inhibitors, but has not clearly found them to be better pain relievers than the older or even nonprescription NSAIDs. Vioxx

(Rofecoxib) and Bextra (Valdecoxib) were taken off the market due to reported cardiac side effects. Over-the-counter NSAIDs include aspirin, Ibuprofen, and naproxen. People can get pain relief from anti-inflammatory medications for pain not caused by inflammation, but the likelihood of relief is decreased.

MUSCLE RELAXANTS

There are numerous types of analgesic medications available that are non-narcotic and non-anti-inflammatory. For muscle-based pain, the muscle relaxants are most important. These include medications such as Soma (Carisoprodol), Flexeril (Cyclobenzaprine), Zanaflex (Tizanidine), Skelaxin (Metaxalone), and Robaxin (Methocarbamol). The benzodiazepines are also used to relax muscles and provide pain relief. They include Valium (Diazepam), Librium (Chlordiazepoxide), Xanax (Alprazolam), and Klonopin (Clonazepam). For muscle pain associated with severe spasm, your doctor might prescribe Lioresal (Baclofen).

NERVE-BASED PAIN MEDICATIONS

For years, neuropathic pain has been the most difficult of all pain triggers to treat. Recently, physicians began using anticonvulsant medications to treat neuropathic pain. Decades ago, anticonvulsant medications were developed to prevent the spontaneous firing of neurons in the brain that can cause seizures. These anticonvulsants raise the threshold necessary to cause seizure activity, in part by lowering the level of central nervous system arousal. These medications also have the effect of decreasing the excitatory cascade and over-sensitization found in the neuropathic pain of many patients. This decreased neuronal activity can decrease pain.

The oldest, commonly used anti-convulsant for pain is Tegretol (Carbamazapine). Newer anticonvulsants for pain include Neurontin (Gabapentin), Zonegran (Zonisamide), Gabatril (Tiagabine), Lamictal (Lamotrigine), and Topomax (Topiramate). Lyrica is a new anti-convulsive type medication and is the only FDA-approved medication for diabetic peripheral neuropathy and post herpetic neuralgia. Depakote (Valproic acid) is a mood stabilizer often used to treat bipolar disorder that is also used by some doctors for neuropathic pain.

Many pain physicians prescribe the older, tricyclic type antidepressants for neuropathic pain such as Elavil (Amitriptyline), Anafranil (Clomipramine), Norpramin (Desipramine), Sinequan (Doxipin), Tofranil (Imipramine), Desyrel

(Trazodone), and Pamelor (Nortriptyline). The tricyclics are also often pre-scribed as a preventative for combined vascular and neurogenic headaches includ-ing migraine and cluster headaches. Doctors also use the triptan family of medications to abort these headaches, such as Maxalt (Rizotriptan), Zomig, (Zolmitriptan) Amerge (Naratriptan), Relpax (Eletriptan), and Imitrex, the origi-nal triptan (Sumatriptan).

ACETAMINOPHEN

Tylenol (acetaminophen) is an over-the-counter medication that is not within any of the classes we have identified. It is a non-narcotic, non-anti-inflammatory in its very own class. This makes it a great medication for infrequent headaches. It also combines with narcotics in an apparently synergistic way that can provide much more pain relief than either does individually. On a long-term basis, the average human body can tolerate about 2,000-3,000 mgs of acetaminophen daily without becoming toxic to the liver. This equates to about 4-6 Extra Strength Tylenol or 3-4 Extra Strength Vicodin. Often the main concern with taking too many narcotics is that they are combined with acetaminophen and a steady, high dose of acetaminophen can be fatal. You should know the milligrams of all ace-taminophen-containing medications and any anti-inflammatory products you are taking.

SCHEDULES OF DRUGS

Prescription drugs are categorized in the United States through the Controlled Substances Act into five schedules based upon the government's perspective of their potential for abuse. At times, a drug's classification is clearly based more on politics than research findings. Schedule 1 drugs are illegal because they have high abuse potential, no accepted medical use, and severe safety concerns.

Schedule 2 drugs have a high potential for abuse and dependence, an accepted medical use, and the potential for severe addiction. They are referred to as the triplicate medications since a copy of the prescription is kept in a national registry in addition to the doctor's office and pharmacy. These drugs include opioids based on high dose codeine, Fentanyl, morphine, and Oxycodone as well as methamphetamine and the barbiturates.

Schedule 3 drugs have a lower potential for abuse than drugs in the first two categories, accepted medical use, and mild to moderate possible addiction. These drugs include steroids, low dose codeine, and Hydrocodone-based opioids.

Schedule 4 drugs have an even lower abuse potential than Schedule 3 drugs, accepted medical use, and limited addiction potential. These include most of the anti-anxiety medications like the numerous benzodiazepines, sedatives, sleeping agents, and the mildest of the opioid type medications like Darvon and Talwin.

Schedule 5 drugs have a low abuse potential, accepted medical use, and very limited addiction potential. These consist mainly of preparations containing limited quantities of narcotics or stimulant drugs for cough, diarrhea, or pain.

USING MULTIPLE MEDICATIONS

Most people with even moderate chronic pain have several of the major pain sources such as inflammation, myofascial pain, tendon or ligament problems, and neuropathic elements. Your pain can be further compounded by inactivity, severe depression, and poor posture, gait, and body mechanics. The most effective medical care requires attacking all these pain triggers for maximal pain relief. As part of your medication regimen, it may be pain relieving for you to take an anti-inflammatory, a muscle relaxant, an anti-convulsant, and a narcotic.

If you are experiencing severe sleeping problems, you may also benefit from taking a sleeping medication, usually one of the older tricyclics. At this point, you would be taking five different classes of medications regularly. This is not at all unusual for someone with multifactoral pain though it may be repugnant to the patient, family, and friends. This is a "cutting edge" multifactoral treatment approach to medication referred to as intellectual polypharmacy by Carl Hess, M.D. in a personal communication (2005). The lowest possible medication doses are used and the synergistic effects of multiple medications are accounted for and even exploited to further reduce pain.

TINCTURE OF TIME

An additional treatment for pain, especially acute pain, is not listed in the W.H.O. ladder of treatments, but is employed by most physicians. It was described to me by my colleague and mentor, John Gurskis, M.D. (1994), as a tincture of time, the physician's secret weapon, which almost by itself heals acute pain. Doctor appointments are typically scheduled two to six weeks apart in the hope that the most recent treatment in conjunction with the passage of time will produce pain relief. Even with chronic pain, the passage of time can help sort out the positive effects of various treatments.

Surgery, therapies, injections, medications, and tincture of time can all be powerful weapons in the battle to eliminate acute pain. They can be absolutely necessary in the treatment of chronic pain and will usually be combined. Multiple factors may be triggering increased chronic pain such as posture, bracing, body mechanics, or lack of sleep. The staggeringly complex interaction between all the sources of tissue damage and the additional pain triggers may make a definitive, specific diagnosis of your pain problem impossible. Often, the best we can do is to identify pain sources and triggers and develop a treatment plan that combats each one of them.

I can use the treatments for acute pain to improve my chronic pain

Insight—I understand the five basic treatments for acute pain that can help my chronic pain.

Commitment—I am committed to assessing these treatments in the context of my pain problem.

Action—I will ask my doctor if she thinks that any of these treatments might help me.

Now—I will advocate for any of the treatments that I think might help me, and one of those treatments is: _____

_____

_____

5

Medical Treatments for Chronic Pain and a New Covenant

The treatment goal for acute pain is simple. Make it <u>go</u> away and I'll be <u>on</u> my way. When your doctor treats the underlying condition and pain effectively, the pain resolves completely, and you are back in the game of life. As we have seen, however, the longer you have wrestled with pain, the more likely it is that your pain will not ever completely go away. This means the longer that you have had pain, the more likely it is that you will not be as fully functional as you were before your pain began.

With chronic pain, the focus of medical treatment needs to shift from cure of the underlying tissue damage and elimination of pain to long-term management of the overall painful condition. In this context, we can think of chronic pain in much the same way we might view chronic illnesses such as diabetes, hypertension, or lupus. We transfer our treatment attention from the underlying condition, e.g., bulging disc or scar tissue, to the pain itself. When your injury or illness becomes stable, pain should become the focus of treatment. You could say that chronic pain becomes the disease or chronic illness that we try to manage effectively.

Several treatments listed on the W.H.O. ladder of pain treatments are more effective and appropriate for chronic pain than for acute pain. Perhaps the negative consequences of the treatment are so great that they would not be attempted with pain that you expected to be cured. If you are receiving these treatments, it is likely that your doctor considers your pain to be chronic, whether or not he has communicated this to you.

EXTENDED RELEASE NARCOTICS TO TREAT CHRONIC PAIN

On the W.H.O. ladder, the lowest rung of treatment that is more appropriate for chronic pain is strong continuous release opioids, including MS Contin (morphine sulfate continuous release), OxyContin (Oxycodone continuous release), Kadian (morphine sulfate continuous release), and Avinza (morphine sulfate extended release), as well as non-oral opioids like the Actiq lollipop and the Duragesic patch, both containing Fentanyl. These medications are normally only prescribed when you have developed a tolerance to the weaker, or instant release medications, and there is the expectation that you will be taking them for an extended period of time, i.e., your pain is chronic.

When you take higher strength, sustained release narcotics over time, you will receive better pain relief with more consistent, less variable dosing and blood serum levels. Common sense tells us that you may not want to treat pain that continues long-term for twenty-four hours a day, seven days per week with a medication that lasts only two to three hours.

BEHAVIORAL AND PSYCHOLOGICAL TREATMENTS OF CHRONIC PAIN

The next rung of treatment on the W.H.O. ladder that is more appropriate for chronic pain than acute pain is behavioral service. In Chapter 1, we described behavioral services as including biofeedback training for posture, gait, and body mechanics; classes in pain coping and rehabilitation; relaxation training; individual psychoeducation; and stress management. These treatments are simply not necessary for the vast majority of patients who have suffered pain for fewer than six months.

Though posture, gait, and body mechanics may be affected with acute injuries, they are not likely to increase your pain significantly yet. Relaxation training is also not necessarily helpful. Psychological education in pain management is effortful, time consuming, and will not be complied with until patients have exhausted almost all other options. However, once other options have been exhausted, and pain is ongoing, patients are far more likely to commit to the hard work inherent in behavioral pain management.

On the W.H.O. ladder of pain treatments, behavioral service precedes surgery when the primary goal of surgery would be pain relief. This makes sense from a medical perspective. Behavioral treatment is much less invasive and less expensive than surgery. Many patients who are surgical candidates but who complete multi-disciplinary pain treatment regimens, including behavioral services, and who commit to the necessary lifestyle changes, subsequently decide not to proceed with surgery because their pain has decreased and their quality of life has improved.

However, many patients with chronic pain who are surgical candidates have the unreasonable hope that surgery will eliminate or dramatically reduce their pain. As a result, they perceive behavioral services and many other treatments as a hoop they must jump through—a process they must complete and fail before they will get the surgery they really need. Their participation in behavioral treatment is a disaster, as these patients tend to be noncompliant and vaguely hostile while creating an unhealthy environment in our rehabilitation and pain classes. It is tragic to admit, but since these patients will eventually undergo surgery anyway, they would probably be better off having the surgery sooner and then three to twelve months later completing behavioral services, if necessary, when they are in a better position psychologically to commit to the work and required lifestyle changes.

THE SPINAL CORD STIMULATOR IN THE TREATMENT OF CHRONIC PAIN

The last two commonly accepted treatments on the W.H.O. ladder are used exclusively for chronic pain. Spinal cord stimulation and indwelling continuous infusion pumps are not considered unless a patient's pain is deemed not only chronic, but also highly likely to be life-long. You may remember that the spinal cord stimulator is an implanted battery with wire leads that sends a warm, vibrating electrical current to the painful area.

If you have moderate to severe pain in one or more arms or legs, which is considered long-term or permanent, you are a candidate for spinal cord stimulation. If that pain is at least partially neuropathic (nerve based), you are an even better candidate for spinal cord stimulation. If the pain is almost entirely neuropathic and radiates from the spine, or is a peripheral or sympathetically mediated pain syndrome, you are a perfect candidate for spinal cord stimulation and may receive tremendous pain relief.

In a personal communication, my colleague, Holly Sata, M.D., (2005) stated, "Spinal cord stimulation is the most powerful and advanced treatment available for chronic, neuropathic pain. All patients with chronic neuropathic pain should be considered for this treatment. Patients need to be educated that this treatment is available and can provide dramatic pain relief and a wonderfully improved quality of life."

You should discuss this treatment with your doctor if you believe you may be a candidate. If she does not think you are a good candidate, and she is not qualified to provide the service, you may want a second opinion from a doctor who is qualified to implant stimulators. The process of determining candidacy for spinal cord stimulation includes a one-week trial period. A small incision is made in the skin near the spine and the leads are inserted. The wires extend outward to a stimulator that is worn on a fanny pack around your waist. The wires are taped down and protected by gauze at the incision site. With the stimulator and wires in place, you can go about your typical activities.

After a week's trial, you will know if the stimulator provides pain relief for you before the device is implanted. If you do not obtain significant pain relief, the stimulator is not implanted. Being able to test drive a treatment without trying it in full is unusual and fairly unique to the implantable devices. There is little permanent risk in completing the one-week trial other than the short-term pain from placement of the trial leads and the possibility of local infection. Jerry Lewis had a stimulator implanted for chronic back and leg pain and became an outspoken advocate for the benefits of stimulation.

Although the stimulator was originally designed for neuropathic pain in limbs, it is being increasingly used for other types of pain in other places. Stimulator leads have been placed at the occipital nerve in the back of the head to treat headache pain. Various types of chest and abdominal pain have been effectively treated with stimulators. Some of the new generation stimulators have up to eight or sixteen leads that can provide pain relief for non-neuropathic pain that extends over a broad area including classic low back or neck pain.

THE NARCOTIC PUMP IN THE TREATMENT OF CHRONIC PAIN

The indwelling infusion pump is another type of implantable device in which a combined battery and reservoir about the size of a hockey puck delivers medication internally. It can be used to treat severe muscle spasms in patients with partial or complete paralysis using an anti-spasmodic medication pumped into the spinal area, typically Baclophen. More commonly, you are a candidate for the pump using narcotic medication if you have chronic, severe low back pain, which is probably permanent.

If you have obtained good pain relief from oral narcotics, you are a good candidate for a lumbar pump. If your pain is grossly compromising the quality of your life, you are an even better candidate. If you only have pain in your low back, you are a perfect candidate and may receive tremendous pain relief. Again, you should discuss this treatment with your doctor. If he believes the treatment is contra-indicated, but does not implant pumps, you may want a second opinion from a doctor who does implant pumps.

As with the spinal cord stimulator, candidates for the "morphine pump" may also receive a trial. Some doctors provide a one-week trial with a small incision made over the spine and a catheter placed so medication can be infused from a pump worn around your waist. This process is identical to that for spinal cord stimulation. Many doctors do not employ a one-week trial pump.

Many physicians give a single narcotic injection into the spinal fluid and assess pain relief over a period of a few hours. Research has suggested that the single injection may be as effective in estimating pain relief from an implanted pump as the one-week trial with much less discomfort and inconvenience.

PAIN MANAGEMENT IS A MEDICAL SPECIALTY

As previously mentioned, pain management is a formal medical specialty with board certification. While pain doctors can treat both acute and chronic pain, my pain physician colleague Richard Paicius, M.D., (2005), noted, "Any patient with chronic pain should seriously consider being evaluated by a pain physician. We are specially trained to provide or coordinate all aspects of chronic pain treatment. Our careers are dedicated to aggressively treating pain and alleviating suffering with the most advanced techniques available."

Pain physicians often provide pain treatment in association with a physician who may be managing the underlying condition. For instance, a patient with severe knee pain who is not an immediate surgical candidate may be better off on a long-term basis having her pain treated by a pain physician rather than an orthopedic surgeon.

If you have severe abdominal pain from gastrointestinal disease such as ulcerative colitis or pancreatitis, you may want a pain physician to treat your pain in addition to your gastroenterologist who is treating the actual disease. If you have frequent, chronic headaches or myofascial pain, a pain physician may be best qualified to treat your pain condition, especially since pain is the real problem.

Most commonly, pain physicians are anesthesiologists, physical medicine doctors, or neurologists. As a rule, anesthesia-trained pain doctors employ more interventions, including all of the injections and the stimulators and pumps discussed above. Physical medicine doctors tend to have more expertise in the musculoskeletal and rehabilitation aspects of chronic pain. Neurologists may have more expertise in neuropathic pain and headache treatment. Most physical medicine doctors and neurologists with expertise in chronic pain also have expertise in many of the injections appropriate for acute and chronic pain, but rarely perform complex injections or implant stimulators or pumps.

Your pain physician's specialty may be less important than his board certification. The original board certification for pain management was provided by the American Board of Anesthesiology (ABA) mainly for anesthesiologists with a specialty in pain medicine. You can access a list of ABA certified doctors at www.abanes.org. Make sure a specialty in pain medicine is documented. The American Board of Pain Medicine (ABPM) also provides board certification in pain management. It is more widely recognized and more open to other medical fields than the ABA board. You can access a list of ABPM certified doctors at www.abpm.org.

The final major board certification in pain is given by the American Association of Pain Management (AAPM) from which I am board certified. This is the only organization that provides board certification for non-physicians and physicians in nontraditional fields. Consequently, you are less certain that physicians from AAPM have been as rigorously trained in pain medicine, as those from the other two boards. A list of AAPM certified doctors is available at www.aapainmanage.org.

WHAT ARE THE TREATMENT GOALS IN PAIN MEDICINE?

With chronic pain, the treatment goals for the patient and the physician are always unique to the patient and the particular condition. But, some general goals can be described. From a patient's perspective, you want to have an improved quality of life. You want to be able to engage in healthy physical, social, pleasurable, and productive activities. You want to have less pain. You want to be happier and suffer less. You want to get on with your life.

Symptoms Related to Pain

From a pain physician's perspective, these goals demand that the multidisciplinary team treat the triumvirate of symptoms, function, and psyche. The pain physician is like the quarterback of the pain treatment team. He can run with certain treatments himself or hand off to other providers for certain treatments, such as manual manipulation, surgery, therapies, and various tests. He coordinates and guides all aspects of your pain care.

Many insurance companies, case managers, and utilization reviewers determine whether they will recommend or authorize a treatment based on the likelihood of long-term pain relief, improved quality of life, or increased function. Many interventions are viewed as failures if they do not achieve permanent benefits. This is insane. Ask a patient if it's worth getting an injection for "only" three months of pain relief, or two months, or one. Ask a patient who has suffered with a severe pain episode for days or weeks if it's worth getting an intervention to get back to their "baseline" level. Pain physicians understand this. They are perfectly willing to provide treatment that is only palliative, as is any doctor who specializes in chronic illness, disease, or injury.

The American Society of Interventional Pain Physicians (ASIPP) is the most widely recognized organization for "anesthesiologists or physicians specializing in pain management, spinal injections, or neural blockade." This is not a board certification, but membership in this organization defines a physician as being interested in using interventional techniques for pain management, a specialty within the field. Moreover, ASIPP published an article detailing evidence based practice guidelines for interventional techniques in pain management (Manchikanti, et al., 2003).

My colleague, Standiford Helm, M.D., noted, "ASIPP guidelines offer detailed commentary as to what criteria should be considered prior to performing any intervention and, for selected procedures, how often various interventions should be delivered and what thresholds should be met to warrant repeating procedures" (2004). This level of standardization and scientific decision-making is what we would all want from the doctor holding the syringe or scalpel.

RESTORING FUNCTION WITH CHRONIC PAIN

Pain physicians also supervise the modalities that aim to improve function, basic activity, and quality of life. These include physical, occupational and water therapies as well as work hardening and vocational rehabilitation. You might be referred for acupuncture, one of the few accepted Eastern approaches to Western medicine. Pain doctors understand the difference between the therapeutic goal of "return to normal function" and the goal of improved function. They can evaluate your work restrictions and disability level, not only from the perspective of tissue-based weakness and injury, but with the knowledge that pain itself is limiting and can produce functional and work-related restrictions.

Psychological Aspects of Chronic Pain

Pain physicians are also very aware of how chronic pain intersects with behavioral and psychological factors. They understand the benefits that patients can receive from behavioral pain services. They know that pain affects quality of life and can lead to distress, frustration, depression, and anxiety. Most pain physicians are highly competent at prescribing medications for depression, anxiety, or sleep disturbance. They understand the reciprocal relationship between psychological adjustment and chronic pain. They know that thoughts and feelings can either inhibit or excite pain signals along the descending tract and open or close pain gates. They realize that behavioral factors can either alleviate pain and increase activity or intensify pain and decrease activity.

Candidly, most pain physicians do not completely understand what goes on in the black box of biobehavioral offices with pain classes, neuromuscular re-education, or individual psychology sessions. But, the patients demonstrate meaningful benefit, which is what the pain doctors know really matters.

WHAT IS THE RELATIONSHIP BETWEEN PAIN AND FUNCTION?

Up to this point, we have been acting as if the treatment goals of decreased pain and increased function were simply complementary and correlated. In fact, with chronic pain, they essentially mean the same thing. I'll explain.

The vast majority of people with chronic pain say that their pain increases with higher activity levels. Virtually all people with pain report that their pain increases with too much activity or with certain types of activity. How much pain you experience at any given moment or in a typical day is powerfully dependent upon the activity level you choose.

In Chapter 3, I asked you to rate your immediate pain, daily variation, and average pain over the past thirty days, all on a scale of 0-100 where 100 is the worst pain you have ever experienced. Your average pain and the numbers your pain varies between on a typical day assume a standard or average level of activity for you throughout an average day and month.

We can rate your typical activity level over the past month (or an earlier month if the past month was unusual) on a scale of 0 (death) to 100, where 100 is your level of activity before your pain problem developed. Take a moment to write down the past month's activity level on the scale of 0-100. Then go back to the pain numbers you produced in Chapter 3 and again write down your average pain over the past month.

My average level of activity over the past month compared to my pre-pain activity was ___/100. My average level of pain over the past month listed in Chapter 3 was ___/100.

Your average pain level over the past month was based on the activity level you listed above. Perhaps you chose a lower activity level of 20-60/100 because higher levels increase your pain beyond what is tolerable. Perhaps your activity level is still rather high because you have to work or care for children which may maintain your pain at a higher level. Whatever the reason for your activity level, your pain is largely dependent on, or a function of, that activity level and vice versa.

Let's say that we have a patient, Jim, who has an average daily pain level of 60/100, with daily variation between 40/100 and 80/100. With that average pain level and variation, his daily activity level averages a 60 on the 0-100 scale. We could ask Jim to help us with an experiment and arbitrarily increase his activity level to 90/100 for a week. We can be 99 percent certain that his average daily pain level will increase from a 60/100 to a 70, 80, or 90/100, most likely to at least an 80. In other words, Jim has an average pain level of 60/100 when his activity level is 60/100 and an average pain level of 80/100 when his activity is 80/100. He has been averaging a 60/100 pain level because he chose a 60/100 activity level. We would probably also discover that his average pain decreased to something like 40/100 if he lowered his daily activity level for a week to 40/100.

If we could help Jim get to the point where his pain averaged 40/100 while he maintained his normal activity level of 60, Jim would say we had decreased his pain and so would we. Then if we artificially had him increase his activity level to a 90/100, his pain would probably only increase from 40/100 to something like 60/100. Good for Jim.

On the other hand, if we could help Jim get to the point where his regular activity level was 90/100 and his pain did not increase beyond his normal 60/100, this would also represent a decrease in his pain, since a 90/100 activity level produced an 80/100 pain level in our previous experiment. Unfortunately, Jim might not be at all happy with this arrangement since the pain he actually experiences in a typical day is unchanged. He might even consider that his treatment had failed. And he would be wrong.

Ultimately, increased activity and decreased pain are different sides of the same coin. With acute pain, we expect that increased levels of function and activity will inevitably be associated with a decreased pain level and vice versa. But, we have seen that the same is not true for chronic pain. Sudden, dramatic increases in activity almost always cause increased pain, at least in the short run.

For a patient with chronic pain, being able to increase activity and have decreased pain is not natural or inevitable as it is with acute pain. You can have less pain with the same activity level, or the same pain with a higher activity level. But, if you want less pain with more activity, that's like getting twice as much pain relief, in perfect balance. It is possible, but it takes a lot of work to achieve, by both doctor and patient. Ignorance about this simple, tragic reality is at the heart of most patients' dissatisfaction with chronic pain treatment and rehabilitation.

A New Contract with Your Doctor

Whether you focus on increasing your activity, decreasing pain, or both, the management of chronic pain requires a fundamental change in the nature of your relationship with your pain doctor. When you go to a doctor for an acute problem, you make an agreement with him, a contract that goes something like this: I will trust you to know and do what is best for me. I will share embarrassing things with you. I will comply with whatever treatments you recommend. I will let you hurt me physically if it will help me in the long run. I will let you touch me in places and do things to me I would not even let my spouse do. And I will even pay you for the privilege, if you will make me well. And the doctor lowers his gaze from the heavens, looks down at the earth and at you, and says, "Okay," or something similar.

However, if you have a chronic illness, injury, or pain, we have established that the doctor cannot make you well. What you do to help yourself is as important, perhaps even more so, than what your doctor does. Remember that 30-70 percent of chronic pain is caused by factors other than tissue damage—mostly things over which only you have control. At 3:00 a.m., when you have not slept at all because of pain, you cannot call your doctor and ask him to sing you to sleep. It's all up to you, and only you.

So your pain doctor needs to sit his Armani-covered butt down and sign a new contract. Part of his role is to educate you about your condition and your options so you can make fully informed decisions. Passive compliance with anything he recommends may not always be helpful. You may have an adverse reaction to a medication, a severe pain increase due to a therapy, or misunderstand his instructions in a way that is dangerous to you or simply wastes your time and money. You need to be actively involved in the development of your treatment plan. Ultimately, you are responsible for the consequences of your treatment failures or gains. At the very least, you and your doctor are partners in the quest for good pain control and pain management.

This changing contract between doctor and patient symbolizes a qualitatively different model in the care of acute vs. chronic pain. In 1991, my mentors Richard Hanson, Ph.D., and Kenneth Gerber, Ph.D., described the changing model in terms of medical management vs. self-management. They referred to the model for treatment of acute pain as Medical Management where the physician is the carpenter and you are the wood. The treatment model for chronic pain is called Self-Management. This acknowledges that success or failure and everything in-between rests with you.

With chronic pain, it is your knowledge, your courage, and your integrity that will make the difference. The pain physician is still extremely important, but you are the carpenter and he is your hammer. As the pain psychologist, I'm not sure where I fit into this metaphor. I'm probably the nails left over after most of the house is built. The point is that our task is to use all the strategies we can, to help you build your house of pain management, referred to in later chapters as your Personal Pain Paradigm. We work for you. You need to work for you, too.

I can use the treatments for chronic pain to improve my pain and quality of life

Insight—I understand the treatments for chronic pain and I understand why increased activity and decreased pain is really the same thing.

Commitment—I am committed to assessing these treatments in the context of my pain problem.

Action—I will ask my doctor if she thinks that any of these treatments might help me.

Now—I will advocate for any of the treatments that I think might help me, and one of those treatments is: _____

_____

_____

6

The Four Stages of Chronic Pain Treatment

Ann was referred to me by her pain doctor immediately after he had completed his initial consultation with her. She was very excited about his treatment plan and encouraged that finally, she had found a competent doctor who really understood her pain. She had seen several other doctors for her pain and she commented that they all just wanted to push medications on her. I inquired about her other doctors and the story spilled out.

After several surgeries on her low back, Ann's orthopedist indicated that he had done all he could and that she needed to "learn to live with it." He referred her to a pain doctor who tried some injections and various medications. She was frustrated that he did not refer her for any diagnostic testing, and after a year, she got a second opinion from another pain doctor. He suggested some diagnostic testing (nerve conduction study and EMG) and various medications. Two years later, having transferred her care to the second opinion doctor, she was still being seen in follow-up for brief monthly appointments during which she mainly received prescriptions for more medication.

She was again frustrated with her doctor's seemingly lackadaisical attitude toward her pain and felt that he was too busy now that his practice had grown. The staff also did not seem as nice to her as they had in the past, and she knew it was time to move on. She then met with another pain doctor who reviewed her case, and suggested new medications that Ann could try, but stated that her doctors had tried almost all appropriate treatments. She felt that she didn't "click" with this doctor since he "just wanted to give me medications" and met with the pain doctor who had sent her to me. He was ordering an MRI and another course of physical therapy with massage. He was also going to try a new type of injection called Botox. She assured me that she was highly motivated to feel better and was encouraged now that she was in a place that was "really going to do something about my pain." Ann was in trouble.

I am a consultant to over a hundred physicians in Los Angeles and Orange Counties including a few dozen pain physicians. Not surprisingly, it turned out that her orthopedist and four previous pain physicians were doctors to whom I consult. I know them to be competent, highly caring physicians and each of them had reached a point of "maintenance" with her, though at different rates. She was enthusiastic with each new physician but as the "bag of tricks" quickly settled into routine follow-up appointments; she became disillusioned and moved on. The physician who had sent her to me had himself lost many patients who had moved on to several of the pain doctors Ann had seen previously.

Clearly, Ann was responsible for her frustration with her doctors and might have moved on to still another doctor in a year or two. Fortunately, she and I had the opportunity to review her case at length and I educated her about chronic pain, realistic treatment goals, and the idea of maintenance care for chronic illness and injury. I further indicated that the primary change that needed to occur was in her accepting the chronicity of her condition and taking responsibility for her rehabilitation. Though I was as gentle and supportive as I could be, she was appalled and angry with me. She accused me of trying to practice medicine and assured me she would be speaking with her pain doctor about me. He reinforced what I had communicated to her since my confrontation and education of her was the main reason he had referred her to me.

Over time, Ann actually invested herself in our multidisciplinary program and committed to the process of feeling better. Three years later, she meets monthly with me and with the referring physician. She is functioning much better with decreased pain. Recently, we completed an end-of-the-year treatment review, and I teasingly reminded her how angry she had been with me after her first appointment. Of course, she was embarrassed, but also proud of how far she had come since then. Congratulations, Ann.

WHAT STAGES DO ALL PATIENTS PROGRESS THROUGH IN CHRONIC PAIN TREATMENT?

Ann had not been taught that there were natural, healthy stages in the doctor-patient relationship. Consequently, each time she approached the final stage, she bolted from the treatment to begin the stages anew. Every patient with chronic pain reaches a point in his or her medical treatment where the doctor's job is primarily to manage and maintain the patient's condition. This is true of almost any chronic illness or injury including diabetes or hypertension. From a physician's perspective, maintenance is the necessary long-term phase of the medical care process for a chronically painful condition. But, this clinical picture can appear very different to the patient.

Discovering

From a patient's perspective, the first stage of chronic pain treatment is Discovering. This is the most hopeful stage, wherein patients and doctors anticipate that there will be a new and more accurate diagnosis that can be so effectively treated that the pain will go away or be permanently reduced. X-rays and MRIs may be used to determine the presence of bone, disc, or joint contributors to pain. EMGs and nerve conduction studies can help assess whether there has been muscle or nerve damage. Some treatments during this stage may help your doctor with differential diagnosis, a term that means the process of deciding between two competing, possible diagnoses.

For instance, if you have neuropathic pain in your arm, your doctor might give you a stellate ganglion injection to determine if you have the sympathetically mediated subtype of neuropathic pain that we discussed in Chapter 2. With chronic pain, differential diagnosis often means determining which pain sources are the strongest contributors to your multifactorial pain and should be the focus of treatment.

Exploring

The second stage of chronic pain treatment is Exploring. Your doctor may try medications, injections, or therapies that you had not previously received. In this stage of care, your doctor may also repeat some treatments that you did try with or without clear benefit.

Another round of physical therapy may be helpful for chronic pain if you and the physical therapist develop a different attitude and treatment goals. We have learned that decreasing pain is not a specific goal of physical therapy, which seeks mainly to increase strength, range of motion, and endurance in a relatively short period. We do know that physical therapy often increases chronic pain, unlike the outcome with acute pain. But we also learned that some physical therapists have expertise in chronic pain. Like you, they know that being able to increase daily physical activity without an increase in chronic pain represents pain relief, since an arbitrary increase in activity almost always increases chronic pain.

You can give yourself permission to proceed very slowly in physical therapy without increasing your pain and be satisfied with only small gains in functional ability and daily activity during your course of treatment. You can use physical therapy mainly as a springboard for continued rehabilitation. You can also learn various exercises that would be beneficial for you to perform long-term on your own. Most physical therapists can give you a list of exercises complete with written instructions and diagrams.

Additionally, at some point in the Exploring stage you may receive behavioral treatments including biofeedback, pain classes, and individual pain psychology. Toward the end of this stage, your doctor reaches the conclusion that virtually every reasonable treatment for your pain condition that is currently available has been tried or ruled out, including implantable stimulators and pumps. You have probably reached the end of the W.H.O. ladder of appropriate pain treatments for you.

Mapping

The third stage of treatment is called Mapping. Your doctor develops a long-term, treatment approach or paradigm designed to keep you as comfortable and functional as possible with some combination of routine medications, sporadic physical therapies, and occasional injections. Your treatment intensity begins to diminish. Most of the modalities like physical therapy or biofeedback either finish or become less frequent. Even your doctor's appointments become less frequent and less complex.

During this stage, you may begin to question your doctor's treatment plan, competence, caring, etc. You may feel the bloom coming off the rose and wonder if a prettier rose can be found elsewhere. But, the development of a long-term treatment paradigm is absolutely necessary and a healthy point to reach in your treatment. It is also the most misunderstood aspect of chronic pain treatment which can produce severe dissatisfaction, anger, frustration, and acting out by patients as they struggle to intensify treatments. What is happening is that your condition is being maintained and the mantle of power for rehabilitation is truly being handed to you.

Building

The final stage of medical treatment is referred to as Building. You can choose to build on the medical care you have been receiving and renew your commitment to self-management. You can help your doctor by researching breakthrough treatments on your own. You can choose to sustain your relationship with your current doctor or pursue the flush of discovery with a new doctor.

As is true for all longer-term relationships, the question becomes "Is he good enough?" You might ask yourself, "Am I confident enough that everything reasonable has been tried? Do I think he is abreast of 'cutting edge' treatments and will try them with me, as they are available? Do I trust him to manage my condition on a long-term basis?" Your answers to these questions should determine whether you stay with your present doctor or move on to another.

Patients are aware of the changes that occur in their medical care during the Mapping and Building stages. Your appointments may become shorter, perhaps going from thirty minutes to ten minutes. They may be scheduled further apart, perhaps from every two weeks to every three months. Your interaction with your doctor may seem more perfunctory. His questioning may be less detailed and he may not follow up your statements with questions about your symptoms. He is clearly no longer interested in getting to the root of the problem, and it can take several appointments before he does much about a report of new symptoms. His main interest may seem to be in refilling your medicine. Not surprisingly, this can be a very disillusioning experience for you as you realize that he and the staff are maintaining you but no longer rallying around you.

WHAT IS THE MAINTENANCE PHASE OF CHRONIC PAIN TREATMENT?

Maintenance is a term with which most pain physicians are quite familiar, but may never discuss with you directly. The process of transitioning to maintenance care is a gradual and subtle one. There is usually no absolute point at which this happens and it is never documented in the medical records. Frequently, this transition is not clearly communicated to the patient, and even the medical providers may realize it only in hindsight some months after it has occurred.

Maintenance or routine follow-up care is much more clearly spelled out in medical-legal cases, such as worker's compensation, personal injury, long-term disability, and social security applications. In these legal settings, the presence of permanent pain and disability needs to be documented and the amount needs to be assessed to determine compensation or entitlement to disability benefits. From a legal perspective, this is often referred to as a permanent and stationary declaration, an awful term that seems to herald the death of hope. But, it does make clear to the patient that medical treatment from this point forward is designed to maintain physical condition and function. We do not anticipate significant improvement in the near future.

Sometimes it is nearly impossible for patients to meaningfully accept the chronicity of their condition and commit to building on the maintenance map of their doctors until there is a dramatic or clear-cut statement made by their medical providers, whether or not they are involved in a medical-legal system. I have treated worker's compensation patients who were clearly never going to assume responsibility for improving their pain condition, if ever, until their "comp" case was settled, or they were at least declared permanent and stationary. Other patients will not commit to self-management until their disability cases or civil lawsuits are finalized. It is hard work to build on your doctor's care by persevering with the hundreds of recommendations made by your multidisciplinary team. Some patients will not begin that work until they have been told that their medical treatment is now mainly for long-term maintenance.

When patients are in the Discovering and Exploring stages of pain treatment at a pain clinic, the program is intense. A total of eight to ten appointments per week is not at all unusual, often making it impractical to continue gainful employment for a time. All your providers are invested in your care. Much of your life and daily activity revolves around treatment for your condition. Considering the physical therapists, biofeedback therapists, chiropractors, pain doctors, psychotherapists, massage therapists, primary care doctors, surgeons, and all their staff, you may be receiving more support and encouragement than at any time in your life. A half dozen or more people are concentrating their expertise, time, and effort to help you feel better. They are deeply concerned about your health and quality of life. Now is the easy time to hope that you will feel better.

During intensive pain treatment, a patient will often complain about the number of appointments he has and how time consuming they are. He may complain that he does not feel like a person anymore, because it seems that everywhere he goes, he is just another patient. He spends most of his day in waiting rooms. He may complain about how some of his providers treat him and describe conflicts with one or more staff members who are rude, don't return phone calls, or are otherwise incompetent. He may talk about how much he is looking forward to the time when his appointments are less frequent and he resumes being a person, not just a patient.

And then you get your wish. All the various therapies end. You see fewer doctors, especially if you are in a medical-legal case. The doctors you do see spend less time, seem less interested, and meet with you less frequently. You are in the Mapping and Building stages. As you go back to being a person, a huge chunk of your support system evaporates and your quality of life may be far worse than you had hoped. Some patients want to stand on the desk and yell, "Wait a minute! Where'd everybody go? I'm not that much better! Come back! I need more of everything!"

This is the critical period in the transition to the Building stage. It is this feeling, at times this near panicky feeling, which may drive you into the waiting rooms of new physicians, who may promise you, if nothing else, a new support system that will "rally 'round" once again. In this stage, you are confronted anew that your condition is chronic and will extend into the future, that your doctor cannot cure you, and that you are left with more pain than you wanted or expected. The losses associated with moving through the Building stage can feel devastating.

Your history of handling losses will affect how you adjust to this stage as will the quality of your support system of family and friends. You can replace the medical providers who cease treating you with non-medical people. For instance, when physical therapy ends, you can begin taking water exercise classes three times a week and develop relationships with the instructor and several group members. If finances allow, you can hire an outside massage therapist. You might join a walking group or make friends through a new type of activity. Ultimately, your ability to adjust to the Building stage and medical maintenance is dependent upon how effectively you are creating healthy and life-affirming experiences and activities.

I can evaluate my medical care in terms of the four stages of chronic pain treatment

Insight—I understand the four stages of pain treatment and the principle of maintenance care.

Commitment—I am committed to moving through these stages as effectively as possible.

Action—I will determine what treatment stage I am in currently and discuss it with my doctor.

Now—I will carefully and deliberately decide if I want to stay with my doctor, move on, or be referred to a pain physician.

7

The Continuum between Pain and Associated Suffering

The word pain comes from the Latin "poena," meaning a fine or penalty. Various medical organizations previously defined pain as "a noxious sensation"—noxious, meaning bad, negative, or unpleasant. Sensation means something physical that happens to you that you can sense, e.g., through sight, sound, touch, smell, or taste. In the early 1990s, the definition of pain changed. This led to a near revolution in how pain was treated. The International Association for the Study of Pain (IASP) now defines pain as "an unpleasant sensory (physical) and emotional (psychological) experience associated with actual or potential tissue damage or described in terms of such damage."

WHY IS IT IMPORTANT TO DEFINE PAIN AS AN EXPERIENCE?

So, pain is an unpleasant physical and emotional experience related in some way to tissue damage. The Latin's might say, "Pain is something that makes you feel like you are being penalized." According to the accepted IASP definition, pain has several aspects. It is unpleasant; people would not seek it out. Pain is both physical and emotional, i.e., it is never just physical or just emotional. Each episode of pain lies somewhere on the continuum from almost purely physical, to almost purely emotional. Pain is something you experience, at times with your whole being.

A noxious sensation is something unpleasant that happens out there, in your environment that you can sense. Nociceptive (stimulus response) pain from the classic stubbed toe might be considered a noxious sensation. You might be able to measure a noxious sensation. An extremely high-pitched noise can be painful and we could measure the pitch and decibel volume of that noxious sensation. If you whacked your head on the lifted hatch of your SUV, we could measure the area of your head that greeted the door and the speed or force with which the contact was made. We could even measure the creativity and loudness of your cursing. But, we could not measure the totality of your painful experience of head whacking. We could not know how much it hurt you.

An experience is an internal event; it happens inside you. You have to make sense of it and integrate it into your other life experiences. In a personal communication, my colleague Marylin Calzadilla, Psy.D., (2005) stated, "Each person's perception of pain serves as the mold that will shape their overall pain experience." From an anatomic perspective, we have learned that pain is processed first in the dorsal horn of the spinal cord and travels up the ascending tract to brain structures responsible for processing thoughts and feelings—the cortex and limbic areas, respectively. The brain processes pain and organizes elements of the painful experience with thoughts and feelings. Further, we learned that pain gates could be opened or closed by the descending tract from the brain through the chemicals produced by thoughts and feelings. Brain processes can regulate and modulate the painful experience.

From an existential perspective, all pain has meaning, and part of the experience of pain, even the intensity of pain, is that meaning. To this extent, pain is purely and utterly subjective. We can try to chop it up into little objective pieces, and we will, but the experiential aspect of pain will remain forever a mystery to everyone but the person involved. In the final analysis, your pain is yours and yours alone.

WHAT ARE THE FOUR QUALITIES OF PAIN?

Any physical and emotional experience like pain has four qualities:

- Sensations

- Thoughts

- Feelings

- Behaviors

Each of these qualities is an integral part of the painful experience. We can discuss them individually, but they form an experience, an integrated whole or "gestalt" that is somehow greater than the sum of its parts.

How Do You Describe the Sensation of Pain?

The sensation of pain has three characteristics. First, there is the type of pain described variously as pressured, burning, sharp, stabbing, throbbing, aching, hot, cold, electric, numbing, squeezing, pressured, lancing, cramping, or tingling. Second, there is the amount of pain, described as mild, moderate, severe, profound, terrible, awful, horrible, excruciating, or agonizing. We might even use the scale of 0-100 or 0-10. Third, there is the variability of your pain described as constant, episodic, sporadic, unchanging, variable, up and down, unpredictable, comes and goes, continual, or 24/7.

What are Pain-Related Thoughts?

There is an infinite array of thoughts associated with a painful experience. I will list some of the most common I have heard over the years.

- It makes me want to die.

- It's all I can think about sometimes.

- It consumes me sometimes.

- I wonder, why me?

- It's so unfair.

- It's punishing.

- I can't think straight.

- I'm forgetful.

- I get confused.

- I am spacey and scattered.

- I just want it to go away.

- I think about the person that did this to me when I hurt really badly.

- Sometimes, I wish my family or friends could spend a day in my shoes so they would know what it's like.

- I wish it would go away.

- I ask God to make it go away.

In addition to the pain itself, there are numerous thoughts about the events that are caused or affected by the pain: marital conflict, financial problems, employment, social activities, etc. These life changes become an integral part of the pain experience, much more powerfully for people with chronic pain than acute pain. In my practice, I see divorce, bankruptcy, legal conflicts, police involvement, suicide attempts, friendships destroyed, passionate hobbies ended, careers splintered, and families blown apart—all caused by the experience of chronic pain.

At times, almost everyone will describe thoughts when they say, "I feel _____." Often, the word that comes after "I feel" is not actually a feeling or an emotion, but a thought. For instance, you might say, "I feel abused." The word "abused" is not a feeling; it is a thought. You think that someone has done something bad to you (abusive) and you do not like it. You might feel angry, scared, or sad about the thought that you were abused. Doomed is not a feeling, either. It is also a thought, though you might say, "I feel doomed." You really mean that you think things will inevitably get worse no matter what you do. Thus, you might feel vulnerable, helpless, hopeless, or sad.

Along these lines, other words that describe thoughts that you might refer to as a feeling include: affronted, beaten down, betrayed, broken, bruised, cornered, crucified, crushed, cursed, devoured, disregarded, flared up, griped, ground down, inept, lazy, long suffering, lost, not caring, over the edge, paralyzed, pressured, provoked, punished, rejected, subjugated, supported, taken advantage of, threatened, tormented, tortured, victimized, and worked up. All these words or phrases are really ideas or beliefs, and not feelings.

What are Pain-Related Feelings?

Pain is certainly associated with thousands of feelings, almost all of them negative, since pain is unpleasant. A short list of pain-filled emotions includes: afraid, aggravated, aggressive, awkward, angry, anguished, annoyed, anxious, apprehensive, ashamed, bored, defensive, dejected, despair, despondent, discontent, disgusted, distracted, distressed, dull, enraged, exasperated, fearful, frantic, fretful, frustrated, furious, gloomy, grief, grim, guilty, hurt, irritated, jealous, jittery, lethargic, lonely, mad, miserable, mopey, mortified, nervous, panic, perturbed, petrified, quivery, repugnant, resentful, resigned, scared, sedated, seething, shamed, silly, solemn, sorrow, stoic, suffering, sympathy, threatened, tight, timid, uncomfortable, unhappy, vexed, vulnerable, weary, worried, and wretched.

What are Pain-Related Behaviors?

Pain is also associated with an almost infinite number of behaviors. We will spend several chapters discussing these behaviors in detail. There are some behaviors that are almost always associated with pain, especially severe pain. People rest, or try to, when they hurt. People "hole up," i.e., they withdraw from others, often preferring to be alone. They moan, wince, limp, go to the doctor, and take medication. They talk about their pain. They do not engage in as many fun activities. Usually, they do not exercise much. They are less physically active.

ASSESSING THE FOUR QUALITIES OF YOUR OWN PAIN

If pain really is an unpleasant experience that has the qualities of sensation, thought, feeling, and behavior, then when people are asked to describe their pain in agonizing detail so other people could understand it, we would expect them to use words, phrases, and sentences that describe all four qualities.

At this time, look at the description list that you generated at the beginning of Chapter 2. Above each word, phrase, or sentence, put the letter that best describes that word or phrase. Use "S" for sensation, "T" for thought, "F" for feeling, and "B" for behavior. Remember that a behavior can be something that you do not do anymore.

Now look at the S's, T's, F's, and B's. Do you have at least one of each? If you have written twelve or thirteen lines worth of words, phrases, or sentences, you probably have several of each of the four qualities. If not, you may have agreed with many of the examples of sensations, thoughts, feelings, and behaviors that I listed in the paragraphs above.

For which of the four pain qualities do you have the most descriptors? For which do you have the least? I have conducted this exercise in every series of pain classes I have taught for over a decade. I have never led a pain class that did not use all four descriptors. That is because the experience of pain truly is comprised of these four qualities.

HOW DO THE FOUR QUALITIES OF PAIN INTERACT WITH EACH OTHER?

Now that we have established that the pain experience consists of sensation, thought, feeling, and behavior, we can look at the relationship between them. Each of the four qualities can affect the others in predictable ways. Figure 7 shows the relationship between pain sensation, thought, feeling, and behavior. Notice that there are arrows connecting each of the four with the other three. This means that a change in one can produce a change in another.

Figure 7: Four Qualities of Pain

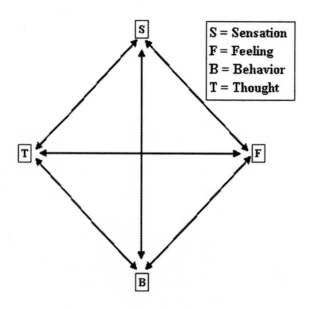

Perhaps the simplest example begins with sensation. Assume that you have low back pain that radiates down your right leg. You step off a curb and land hard with a jolt. Immediately, the pain in your low back intensifies, your legs buckle, and you feel pain in your left leg. Oh my God! What just happened? Did I finally blow out the other disc? Did I screw up the nerves going into my left leg? Dammit! Why does this stuff always happen to me? Are things going to get worse? The pain in your left leg quickly goes away but your low back is on fire. Scared and discouraged, you go home, grab the heating pad, and obsess about whether or not you should make an appointment with your doctor or go to the emergency room.

In this scenario, you have the sudden sensation of increased pain in your back, so we begin at Figure 8 with sensation. The thoughts come fast and furious about what catastrophes the pain could be coming from, so the arrow moves down and toward the left from sensation to thought.

Figure 8: Sensation-Based Progression through Qualities of Pain

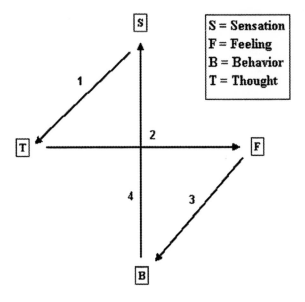

These thoughts produce feelings of fear and anger, so the arrow moves horizontally to the right from thought toward those feelings. Now you go home and grab a heating pad, which moves the arrow down and left from feeling toward behavior. The heating pad warms and loosens up the muscles you strained which decreases your pain sensation and moves the arrow straight up from behavior and returns to sensation. In this example, we could consider that the triggering event was actually the behavior of stepping off the curb, which triggered the increased sensation of pain and led to the thoughts, feelings, and other behaviors.

As another example with a different starting point, Sally was a patient of mine who almost always had worse pain on the weekend. It was early in my career and I decided it was due to some psychological factor—maybe she was less guarded emotionally on the weekend. But, when we were discussing the S, T, F, B qualities in pain class, she described with new insight why her pain was worse on weekends. She said that throughout a typical week (Monday through Friday), she was much less active than she had been before her injury when she worked full time. By Friday afternoon, she was disgusted and ashamed of her inactivity the previous four days and subsequently did some intense, heavy labor—mopping the floors, cleaning the oven, or doing all of the laundry. By Saturday morning at the latest, her pain was "lit up like a Christmas tree" and the pain remained at an increased level for most of the weekend.

In this situation, Sally began with a thought, "I'm a slug." This led to feelings of guilt and shame, which in turn resulted in a behavior—heavy labor that produced a severely increased sensation of pain.

In Figure 9, we start with Sally's original thought, then go right with the arrow to feeling, then down, and left to the behavior, and then straight up to the sensation. Note that you can begin with any of the four qualities and it will inevitably affect the other three.

Figure 9: Thought-Based Progression through Qualities of Pain

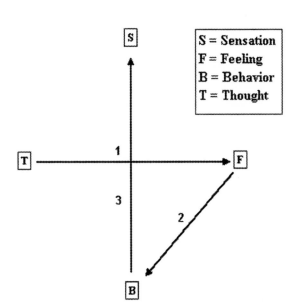

What is the Difference between Pain and Suffering?

Although all four qualities are an integral part of the pain experience, for practical and treatment purposes, we refer to the sensation of pain as pain and the thoughts, feelings, and behaviors as suffering. According to the information already presented and the report of almost every pain patient with whom I have ever worked, the suffering component of pain (reflected in thoughts, feelings, and behaviors) is much greater with longer-term, chronic pain than it is with shorter-term, acute pain. This is another way of explaining the fact that on average 80 percent of acute pain is based upon real or potential tissue damage (20 percent due to other factors) and on average only 30-70 percent of chronic pain is based upon tissue damage (30-70 percent due to other factors).

Previously, we discussed that chronic pain was often increased by central and peripheral sensitization and the chronic hyper-excitation of A-Delta and C-pain nerve fibers. These factors are rarely involved in acute pain and partially explain why chronic pain is more affected by factors other than the original tissue damage. Now we can complete the picture and acknowledge that included in the factors affecting chronic pain is the impact of suffering caused by thoughts, feelings, and behaviors.

You can conceptualize this discussion in terms of the pain gate model. Thoughts, feelings, and behaviors can either open or close pain gates. They can turn the pain volume either up or down. This happens at multiple levels including electrical and biochemical.

If you feel momentarily distracted from your pain, you might think of this as "mind over matter." In fact, there are biochemical and electrical changes occurring including increased production of inhibitory chemicals, increased firing of inhibitory neurons, and closing of pain gates that are literally decreasing your pain sensation. Mind over matter is actually matter over matter.

We can appreciate that the four qualities of pain are different facets of the same prism. We know that pain sensation and suffering affect each other and that each is always a part of the pain experience. Based on the IASP definition of pain, we discussed a continuum of physical and emotional experience with all pain episodes somewhere between almost purely physical and almost purely emotional. At this time, we can substitute the term "suffering" for the emotional experience. Thus, we can also think of pain and suffering as on a continuum determined by the relative contributions of pain sensation and pain suffering toward the global pain experience.

Nearly pure sensation is on the far right of the continuum; nearly pure suffering on the far left; and a solid mixture of both somewhere in the middle. In the old Star Trek television series, imagine the unemotional Mr. Spock receiving an injection. "Dr. McCoy, you're not doing it right. Let me help." There's not much suffering there, so this experience is on the far right of the pain-suffering continuum. Now imagine an out-of-control, screaming, crying, hiding, snotting four-year-old getting that same injection. This is almost pure suffering, so it's on the far left of the continuum.

The longer you receive medical treatment for pain, the more suffering naturally becomes a part of your pain experience. I do not mean to equate you with a snotting four-year-old, but people with chronic pain suffer more than do people with short-term pain. Your pain doctors know this and the longer you hurt, the more they need to estimate where on the pain-suffering continuum you usually fall.

The truth is that if you are on the far left end of suffering, some medical treatments will not help you that much. If you are on the far right end of pain sensation, some psychological treatments will not help you that much. Mr. Spock is not going to need three sessions with a pain psychologist to prepare him for his injection. Your doctor's perception of where you are on the pain-suffering continuum must, and will, affect the recommended treatments, and how they are delivered.

Your position on the pain-suffering continuum is not singular or static. Sensation, thoughts, feelings, and behaviors are fluid. They change continually and always vary from event to event. Thus, the impact of suffering on pain sensation and your place on the continuum will be different in any given situation.

I will give a common example. Perhaps the muscle-based or myofascial aspects of your pain are strongly influenced by thoughts, feelings, and behaviors. If you are highly anxious, you may tense up and make your real pain much worse. In the context of myofascial pain, you tend to be on the left end of suffering. On a long-term basis, you may obtain more benefit from a course of biofeedback using neuromuscular re-education and relaxation training than you would by using long-term muscle relaxants. Conversely, the nerve-based aspects of your pain may be minimally influenced by your thoughts, feelings, and behaviors. For neuropathic pain, you tend to be on the right end of pain sensation. Behavioral treatments would be less beneficial, but anti-convulsants might provide excellent pain relief.

You know there is more misery associated with hurting for a decade than there is for a day. You may find yourself responding to this common sense statement with a resounding DUH! This is obvious to anyone who has been hurting for a long time. It occupies your thoughts, produces all kinds of negative feelings, and changes hundreds of behaviors, affecting the very fabric of the way you live your life. It can change your basic identity—challenging your sense of who you are to the very core.

HOW DOES THE MEANING OF PAIN AFFECT YOUR SUFFERING FROM PAIN?

In any situation, the meaning you give to a pain episode will strongly affect your position on the pain-suffering continuum. Let's look at three examples, beginning first with the pain of childbirth. This is the most catastrophic pain a woman may well ever experience. It is compared by some to severe kidney stones, cluster migraine headaches, or a broken femur. Bill Cosby said, "Imagine pulling your bottom lip up over your head." But, many women will say, "It wasn't that bad. It could have been worse."

When my wife said exactly those words about the birth of our daughter, Leah, I joked and told her, "You must not have been there. I was, and it really was that bad." But, the relevant fact is that the meaning of childbirth pain is glorious. For many women, the experience and the memory of the pain is transcended by the wonder and awe of delivering a new life, her child, into the world. The pain is remembered as bad, but it created a life-altering, wondrous child that changes Mom's identity and life forever, in a positive way—at least until the child becomes a teenager.

Contrast this with the pain from end stage brain and spine cancer. The pain is reflective of a malignant process that is eating away at the body, consuming it from within. We can expect the pain and decay to worsen, other medical problems to pile up, and the misery to steadily increase. The only true release is death. The meaning of the pain is the crystalline reflection of decay and death—a terror so great, we can only write about it if we have never known it, suffering so great and the body so ravaged that death can become a welcome friend.

Now, contrast the pain of childbirth and terminal cancer pain with benign, chronic pain. There is no specific meaning of chronic pain. Yes, the body has been injured and there is residual tissue damage, but we already knew that. There is no positive outcome from the pain, nor does it signal steady deterioration and decay. It is neither fatal nor glorious. It will not kill you unless you decide to kill you. It just is.

We might use many of the same sensation words to describe these three examples of pain, like cramping, tearing, horrible, or excruciating. But, the meaning of these three examples and the associated suffering defined by thoughts, feelings, and behaviors is extremely different. They are simply not the same experience though the sensations may be similar.

People with chronic pain know this in their hearts, even if they cannot completely put it into words. This is why they blanch when someone says, "I know how you feel. I had back pain once." That possibly well-intended comment is ignorant at best, and offensive and hostile at worst. You cannot accurately equate the suffering from a brief episode of steadily decreasing pain that you know will go away, with the wildly fluctuating pain that you know in your heart probably will not go away.

If you have chronic pain, you know that only other people with chronic pain "get it." Even pain doctors and pain psychologists cannot completely "get it" if they do not have it. They are also well intended but a little ignorant. Perhaps not freakin' clueless, but a little ignorant, nonetheless.

We have discussed the difference between acute and chronic pain. We summarized the treatment for acute pain as medical management and the treatment for chronic pain as self-management. Now, we can clarify that with chronic pain, medical management is still vitally important for the treatment of the sensation aspect of the pain experience. You can still benefit from all the tools in the pain doctor's bag. But, the critical element in your rehabilitation is self-management, especially for the suffering aspect of the pain experience.

You have seen that by changing your thoughts, feelings, and behaviors, you can suffer either more or less. You can speed inhibiting chemicals and nerve impulses down the descending tract from the brain through the dorsal horn and decrease your pain. By changing your thoughts, feelings, and behaviors, you can also change the sensation of pain, perhaps from burning to cramping, or from excruciating to "tolerable." The path to sensation does not begin and end with sensation, but can begin with thought, feeling, or behavior. It is in this way, and for this reason, that you can learn to exercise control over your sensation of pain.

Many years ago, I worked with Mary, a very difficult patient. She was angry, belligerent, and noncompliant. She abused her narcotics and drank copious amounts of alcohol. She blamed us for everything that went wrong in her treatment and her life. Her detoxification from narcotic medication and alcohol was necessary but truly horrific with vomiting and hallucinations. She suffered terribly, and made it her goal to have us share in her suffering (otherwise, she was quite sweet). In spite of all this, or maybe because of it, I came to like her and I think we achieved a mutual respect.

At the end of Mary's formal pain program, I conducted the exit interview and asked her to rate her average pain again on a scale of 0-100. True to herself, she declared, "You know I hate that numbers crap, Doc. I don't know if I have less pain or not. I just know it doesn't bother me as much and that's good enough for me." Well, that was good enough for me, too, Mary. So, now, let's focus on you, the reader.

I can use the difference between pain and suffering to create less of both

Insight—I understand the four qualities of the pain experience: Sensation, Thought, Feeling, and Behavior.

Commitment—I am committed to suffering as little as possible.

Action—I will begin to pay attention to pain related thoughts, feelings, and behaviors.

Now—I will document some of my unhealthy thoughts, feelings, and behaviors in my TAAP journal.

8

The Terrible Truth about Coping with Pain

The terrible truth about coping with pain is that people cope with pain the way they have coped with other aspects of their lives. Since Shakespeare, psychologically minded people have known that the best predictor of future behavior is past behavior. When people develop a pain problem, they bring to their pain a system of coping, a hierarchy of strategies for living that they have learned from previous life situations.

People in pain do not suddenly morph into a different person, with a completely different coping style, born of a completely different history. Rather, they apply the same hierarchy of strategies to pain that they have applied to every other life situation. People who have coped badly with life are probably going to cope badly with pain. Conversely, people who have coped well with life will probably cope well with pain.

THE SEVEN LIFE CHOICES THAT CREATE A PAIN-RESISTANT PERSONALITY

In the context of the terrible truth, we need to evaluate effective strategies for life management so that we can apply them to the specific situation of pain management. These strategies are founded on the choices you make on a regular basis that drive the events in your life.

There are seven basic choices we make that determine the direction and character of our lives. These choices are the loom from which our personality is woven. A history of making these choices effectively creates the tapestry of a pain resistant personality, one that minimizes and copes well with physical and emotional pain.

The pain-resistant personality is born of a pattern of choices that improves quality of life and decreases pain. From an anatomic viewpoint, the pain-resistant personality style applied successfully closes pain gates by impeding excitatory signals and speeding inhibitory signals down the dorsal horn.

The seven life choices that comprise the pain-resistant personality are hierarchical in importance, and are associated with corresponding thoughts, feelings, and behaviors. The choices are:

1. Honesty

2. Courage

3. Independence

4. Creativity

5. Planning

6. Initiating

7. Persevering

Every strategy for life or pain management can be understood as subsumed within one of these seven choices or steps. Effectively living with chronic pain is also the product of a pattern of healthily making these seven choices. Ineffective pain coping is the inevitable consequence of failing to consistently make these seven choices in a healthy way. Unfortunately, your coping efforts can be derailed by failure at any one of these steps, although the earlier in the hierarchy you fail, the worse the consequences.

As a rehabilitation and pain psychologist, I should demonstrate these seven choices to my patients. I should be honest with them and courageously deal with tough issues, even those that might make them angry with me, like noncompliance. I must be independent and not simply a mouthpiece for their physicians. I should be creative in planning their treatment and flexible with changes as perceived obstacles appear. I must initiate the plan that I develop each step of the way. And I need to persevere.

I want my patients to see me as relentless in my purposeful efforts to help them feel better, even when they tire and do not feel relentless. I want them to feel my passionate belief in the ability of behavioral services to decrease their pain. I want them to know the power of self-management as it transforms their lives. I should be a role model for these seven choices. You can probably imagine that this is not always well received. While I get cards and letters testifying to the glory that is my work, in a twenty-five-year career I have also been assaulted, spit on, screamed at, threatened, had my tires slashed, and had a book thrown at me (not even one I had written).

High quality behavioral pain management is not simply supportive psycho-therapy. It is not just some ephemeral, feel-good gauze that comforts you, or makes you feel better about yourself, simply because you draw breath. It is educational, intense, important, and difficult. Patient's emotions run high and the consequences are extreme, either improved quality of life and a measure of contentment, or life-long misery and suffering. It is not a game. You owe me nothing but to pay your bills on time. I owe you the best I have during every single appointment, and you owe yourself the same.

Honesty about Life and Pain

Life choices begin with honesty. This is not simply about telling the truth to others. It is choosing to see the world as it is. Not the way you want it to be or fear it will become in the future. Not the way it was in the past. The way it is…now. You need to be honest about the people around you and the environment in which you live. But, you must be honest with yourself first and always; honest about whom you are, especially your strengths and weaknesses.

I have been reasonably athletic my whole life. I can still lift weights and jog for a couple of miles a few times a week. But, honesty dictates admitting that I am also a middle-aged man with two bad knees, an angry sacroiliac joint, and a right shoulder that is convinced I should not have pitched baseball in my youth. Spicy foods tear up my stomach and my doctor says my prostate could be used as a life raft. I am what I am.

Chronic pain is terrible. It wreaks havoc in almost every area of your life. The difference between who you were and who you have become can be staggering and demoralizing. But, being honest means accepting that your pain will remain indefinitely. It means being realistic about which activities are healthy and which are not. It means taking a long hard look at your life, and recognizing how it has changed and must change further. It means being honest with the people in your life. It means being honest about what you want from life, medical treatments, and the world around you. You cannot hope to cope well with pain if you are dishonest about your pain sensation, thoughts, feelings, or behaviors.

Over the years, I have seen patients deny the long-term nature of pain that has lasted for years and resisted numerous medical interventions. These patients keep expecting to feel better from the next medical treatment, and give themselves permission to place their lives on hold until they feel good again. They have a vague idea of all the things they want to do after their pain goes away or improves dramatically. Unfortunately, they need to stop putting their lives on hold, and re-engage in activity in order to feel better, regardless of their medical treatments.

Some patients blame their doctors that their pain has not been eliminated. Some convince themselves and others that they will do anything to feel better, when what that really means is, "I will let a doctor do anything to me that she wants, and that the insurance will pay for, but don't ask me to help myself." This allows some patients to continue being undisciplined and noncompliant, while not taking any responsibility for their lack of progress.

Patients may deny that they are noncompliant with treatment because they do not like the way "noncompliant" sounds. Often, they believe that if they have a good reason for being noncompliant, that it is the same as being compliant. It isn't. Being noncompliant is not always bad, as we will discuss later, but being dishonest about it is. Some patients deny that they take more medication than is prescribed, and then they just cannot understand how they run out early.

Some patients severely exaggerate or minimize their reported activity level. Some spend years battling desperately for social security disability, long-term disability, 100 percent disability through worker's compensation, or pursue a private injury lawsuit, and still convince themselves that they are committed to being as functional as possible. In a later chapter, we will explore why this is impossible.

Many patients convince themselves they have a high pain tolerance when they really do not. About 80 percent of my patients are convinced they have an extremely high pain tolerance. Statistically, this is impossible. About 50 percent of my patients must have a pain tolerance below average. Only about 50 percent could have a pain tolerance above average, and fewer still could have an unusually high pain tolerance. Previously, we discussed that because of sensitization and "wind up," people in long-term pain are likely to have biochemically reduced pain tolerances.

Facing Your Life and Your Pain Courageously

Courage is the second choice imperative for effective living. You are confronted daily with situations that are stressful or scary. It is absolutely vital that you create a history of attacking scary, difficult, challenging situations head on, all out, without reserve. The greater the fear, the more important it is to challenge it. Every time you avoid a scary situation, you reinforce avoidance as a primary coping strategy. You learn that you cannot count on yourself to manage your own fear. If you know you are a coward, you cannot trust that you will confront anything stressful in the future. Anxiety and dread will increase as your activities become ever more restricted to the easy and familiar. On the other hand, if you historically confront stress and fear head on, you can trust that you will continue to do so.

In a personal communication, my colleague, Andrew Merritt, M.D., described the issue of pain quite simply when he commented, "As part of the human condition, pain is the single greatest physical, psychological, social, and emotional challenge that humans face. The tragedy of chronic pain allows this challenge to go on indefinitely and unrelenting." (2005) Well said, Dr. Merritt.

Facing chronic pain takes more courage than facing almost anything else. In my book, *Stepping Stones: Ten Steps to Seizing Passion and Purpose*, I stated, "I have been left awestruck and speechless by the courage, integrity, and dignity of people facing challenges I can only imagine. I have been humbled and tearful at the loving compassion and profound wisdom of those whose lives gave them every right to lash out at anyone who came near." But, I have also seen tremendous cowardice in the face of pain and its spawn.

I have seen people who are tired of working, use pain as an excuse to stop working. Some people do not tell their doctors what they want or need, for fear of being criticized or otherwise punished. Some people allow their lives to be consumed by medical treatments, or fighting doctors or insurance companies so they do not have to face the real world.

People in pain may become restricted to the house or bed, because they face fewer demands there. It is less scary in bed. Some people will refuse to engage in a new pain management behavior simply because they have never done it before. Some may allow their spouses to speak for them during doctor's appointments because they fear making mistakes or being criticized. Other people use pain as an excuse not to leave catastrophically unhealthy living situations or marriages.

It is not fashionable or politically correct to talk about courage as a behavior or choice necessary for mental health or effective coping. Self-help books and psychotherapists are much more comfortable spending our time and money attempting to make us understand why and how we became cowards in certain situations rather than changing that behavior or confronting poor choices. Ultimately, acting courageously is always a choice often done in a setting where no one else will know or care how brave you have been. But you will know and you should care.

Commitment to Independence through Life and Pain

The third choice that guides effective living is independence. This is the willingness to travel some parts of your life journey alone. It is the willingness to make your own decisions, your own mistakes, to be responsible for your successes and your failures. True independence means having an identity separate from the people or things around you. You need to be comfortable alone, with just you and your thoughts. You need to believe that no one else is responsible for your happiness or your misery. Just you.

Independence is tougher when you hurt. You may feel weak, damaged, and vulnerable. It is the most natural thing in the world to want others to take care of you when you are sick or in pain. One of the major benefits of being married is being cared for when you are feeling bad, physically or emotionally. But, I have seen independence maintained in the face of extraordinary medical conditions and pain, such as single moms with severe pain who work full time, raise kids, and volunteer in school. And I have seen patients with moderate pain surrender all responsibility to their spouse or others, becoming in every sense of the word, another child.

Instead of giving you a list of dependent behaviors, I want you to meet Susan, a 33-year-old Fibromyalgia patient who came to her initial consultation with me accompanied by her husband. They entered the room with his hand cupping her elbow to help support her weight. He frantically searched for an appropriate chair and made a beeline for the recliner we use for relaxation training. He settled her in and reclined her fully, moving his chair over by the recliner. After stroking her hair, he fired up his laptop computer as we began talking.

Susan sat motionless in the chair, as if she were paralyzed. Her husband answered most of my questions as he had proudly stored all of the relevant information in his laptop. Susan did not remember the names of her last doctors, what medications she was taking, or what treatments she had received, because as she said, "He takes care of all that stuff." Her husband even estimated her pain severity on a scale of 0-100.

I discovered that Susan spent twenty-three of twenty-four hours each day in her bed, which her family had moved into the living room, and around which the entire household was organized. Her mother had become quite adept at caring for her until her husband came home from work, which was increasingly part time. He did all the domestic chores or paid to have them done. She did not have any idea about their finances or anything related to the future. She was struggling unsuccessfully to get qualified for Social Security benefits. Describing that process was the only time she showed any real emotion during the appointment.

I learned that this couple had not been sexual for the past six of their seven years of marriage, and both assured me that this was not a problem since neither of them wanted children. Susan's husband gently communicated to me that, while their current pain doctor had wanted them to see me, they would need to ask me some questions to be certain that I understood Fibromyalgia and was qualified to work with them. In particular, they wanted me to understand that any movement at all hurt her, including talking very much. They were deeply disappointed to learn that my primary treatment goal would be to get her out of bed and improve her pain and activity. They wanted to focus on helping her extended family adjust to her condition and help take care of Susan.

I did not believe I would ever see them again and, indeed, they did not return for treatment. I truly believe they both had what they wanted. Susan chose to relinquish all independence and became totally dependent on her husband. He chose to be married to a four-year-old. I still feel sad whenever I think about that couple.

Permission to Be Creative toward Life and Pain

Creativity is a silent, but important life choice. To be creative is to create, to bring something into being. For our purposes, it means trying novel approaches to life and problem solving—what business types call "out of the box" solutions. It means committing to learning, stretching, reaching, and growing as a person. You do not have to restrict yourself to the familiar. You can give yourself permission to change your coping hierarchy, and to try new things. Learning pain management will take you out of your comfort zone. You will need to give yourself permission to try all kinds of new, weird things to manage your life better with pain in it. You can imagine a world that is better than what you have. Even if you fail, you learn.

Creativity and hope are inexorably linked. Before you can set goals and plan for the future, you need to be able to imagine a better, changed future. Ultimately, pain management is just life management for a person in pain. You need to be creative and try new approaches. You can explore new ways of coping with pain, communicating with others, or simply living life.

Drop the censor, the voice that says, "That won't work," or "I've tried that before." You can realize that some of the things you have learned about pain are wrong. You can feel better. You can have less pain. You can learn to do more and improve your life. But you will need to be creative, to do less of the same old, same old and more of the new. And the new is always scary. Fear is the enemy of creativity and courage is its ally.

Planning Life Even with Pain

If creativity is the art of coping with life, then planning is the science that helps you reshape it. Effective living is not simply reacting to, or coping with, the world as you find it, but proactively changing it to better suit your needs. This means planning and lots of it. You need to plan for old age, retirement, when the kids go to school, emergencies, education, health, and prioritizing your daily activities. This goes against the new age books that champion "living in the now." This is only healthy if you have planned for your short, medium, and long-term future while actively engaged in achieving your goals. Then you get to sit on a beach and enjoy the now.

Planning and effective pain management are practically synonymous. If you just "take each day as it comes and do what I can," then you will be accepting a miserable day and doing very little. Planning takes you from reacting to your painful life as it is, to proactively making it better. You can plan physical, social, pleasurable, and productive activities. You can plan how to handle the unexpected crises that come up, some of which are not completely unexpected or a crisis. Like all good science, planning should be written down, preferably in your TAAP journal. You can know that you are captaining your own ship rather than letting the pain chart your course.

Planning is incorporated into the integrated approach of self-management referred to as your Personal Pain Paradigm. A paradigm is a philosophical or theoretical framework consisting of theories, laws, generalizations, and experiments. Your characteristic approach to living is a paradigm, born of theories and rules about how the world works and should work. Each time you perform a behavior and receive feedback from the world, you have conducted an experiment and made generalizations about it. Your pain paradigm is the application of ideas, strategies, and experimental behaviors related to pain and the conclusions you reach about them.

The planning involved in the development of your Personal Pain Paradigm is the confluence of strategies you have thought, read, heard, and tried. It guides your behavior. Though your long-term goals may remain the same, your short-term goals and strategies will evolve as they are confronted by success or failure in the real world. Truly effective planning is a continuous process molded by the outcomes of behaviors. We noted previously that your Personal Pain Paradigm is not simply a strategy for your own coping, but includes the triumvirate of what your doctor can do for you, what you can do for yourself, and what you can do for your doctor.

Every day I see people champion their own refusal to plan, and to establish a healthy Personal Pain Paradigm for daily living. They will say, "My wife does all the planning." They may lead unhealthy, unstructured lives and say, "I can't plan anything because I don't know how I'm going to feel." Yes you do. You will have pain and feel bad. You can base your planning on having pain and feeling badly. If you need to alter your plans, you can do so, but make healthy plans. If you do not, you will do less and feel worse than you would have otherwise.

Initiating Your Plan

Initiating seems to be the most difficult of the seven basic life choices for many people. You create and plan courses of behavior based on honesty and courage that satisfy healthy independence. Then, you need to initiate the plan. Some call this the divine spark, the "let there be light" moment, the "Eureka" event. In old books and scriptures, it was the moment of "and it came to pass." They never told you how it came to pass, just that it did.

There are strategies for initiating activity. Most important is to make the initial behavior as easy as possible. You may need to remove obstacles or excuses. It is helpful to have your plan broken down into small steps. Reminder notes may be helpful, as well as keeping the consequences of not initiating the plan or a change in front of you. It is also important to keep the long-term goal firmly in mind, with a clear understanding of how that first step will initiate the process of healthy change and goal achievement.

Initiating a behavior that you have planned is so much harder when you have chronic pain. Because of pain, stress, and exhaustion, doing anything new or different can feel larger than life. It can be hard enough to keep putting one foot in front of the other. Anything extra can feel overwhelming. Sometimes, the behavior you have planned simply never reaches a high enough level of importance, or becomes a priority above all others.

Let's meet Joe, a 45-year-old, divorced, regular guy. He has a mild problem with low back pain, and a little shoulder and knee arthritis. Joe lives alone, has managed to get himself disability retirement, and he has friends with whom he spends some time. He plans every day to exercise at the gym since exercise always makes him feel better. But he also likes staying on the couch, watching television, and eating sweets. It's less work. First weekly, then monthly, Joe would attend his appointment with me and explain why he had not exercised that week. For over a year, I tried everything in my psychologist's bag to get him to exercise. Each week he would come in, disappointed with himself, and with me, because, once again, whatever I had tried had failed. He still had not exercised.

Maybe Joe was too depressed to exercise. Maybe he had some deep-seated fear of exercising. Maybe exercise was too demanding. Maybe not. In truth, Joe had always been a reactive, unambitious, relatively lazy guy, who had spent his life taking the easy way out of everything. He dealt with what the day presented and did not think much about tomorrow. Joe had never been a big planner or persevered with much of anything in his life, including exercise, and he didn't really want to start now. I think each day, he was perfectly comfortable on the couch, or hanging with his friends. It was only in the evenings, or when he had appointments with me, that he considered what he thought he "should" be doing. Kind of in the same way, I occasionally think I should learn Spanish because I live in Southern California, but it's so much work, and there's always something more important to do, like watching reruns of Bonanza.

Persevere With a Healthy Life and Pain Management

Perseverance is the least sexy of the seven basic life choices. Yet, most goals in life that you want to achieve require some perseverance. Usually, the more important the goal, the more you have to persevere to achieve it. And sticking-to-it is only helpful in the service of a carefully crafted plan to achieve a clearly defined goal. Perseverance for the sake of persevering, or stubbornness, or unwillingness to try a fresh approach is not healthy.

Our culture does not seem to encourage perseverance. Much of the feel-good literature and get-rich-quick schemes are based on the premise that you can reach important goals without having to persevere, which usually means not having to work hard.

People who persevere in life are much more likely to persevere with strategies for pain management. My brother, Eric, has persevered in many ways throughout his life. He taught me the phrase "failing upward." He injured his back skiing about five years ago and spent several months in rehabilitation. Recently, I learned that even though he is now pain free, he has continued to do the daily stretching and strengthening exercises that he learned in physical therapy to prevent another episode. I would call that perseverance. Most of us forget to take the antibiotics after we start feeling better.

People in pain who are not used to persevering will struggle with the routine and mind-numbing regimen that may be necessary to manage chronic pain well. Trying to "keep busy," trying to "maintain a positive attitude" or "not dwell on it," and trying to "rest when I need to," sound like good ideas. But they do not qualify as perseverance in the service of a carefully crafted plan of self-management, to achieve a clearly defined goal, pain relief.

The above seven life choices are unforgiving. You can deceive other people. You may even be able to deceive yourself. However, you will suffer the consequences of your deception until you commit to making good choices and act on that commitment. It is true that people tend to deal with pain the way they have dealt with other life experiences. But, with your new insights, you can address some of your weaknesses and lean on some of your strengths.

You can choose to weave the tapestry of a pain-resistant personality. Such a personality certainly helps you cope better with chronic pain. More importantly, the pain-resistant personality actually decreases pain by increasing the inhibitory pain signals coursing down the dorsal horn from the brain.

Spend some time thinking about the seven basic choices, and think about how you made them before you had pain. How do you make these choices now that you have pain? What are some areas in which you need to change? You will receive hundreds of suggestions in the following pages.

Being mindful of the seven life choices can help me manage pain more effectively

Insight—I understand that how I make the seven choices can create a pain-resistant personality.

Commitment—I am committed to making these choices better than I have in the past.

Action—I will begin evaluating my life and daily activities in terms of the seven choices.

Now—Today I will make one of these choices more effectively than I have previously, and that choice is: _____

_____

_____

9

How to Minimize Pain-Related Behaviors

We have demonstrated that pain includes the four interdependent qualities of sensation, thought, feeling, and behavior. We have identified the seven choices that affect your pain, suffering, and self-management. We have described your global approach to pain relief as your Personal Pain Paradigm. We will continue our discussion with the behavioral choices that affect pain. These choices include specific pain behaviors as well as more global physical, social, pleasurable, and productive activities.

WHAT ARE PAIN BEHAVIORS?

Pain behaviors can be loosely defined as those behaviors that you engage in that communicate to other people that you hurt. We are not saying that you always perform these behaviors to communicate that you have pain; just that these behaviors suggest to others that you are hurting or have a limiting medical condition. Although most of these behaviors are a natural response to pain, they should be minimized as much as possible. In one way or another, each of the following pain behaviors is unhealthy and either increases pain, decreases function, or both.

WHAT IS THE PAIN MASK?

The most ubiquitous of pain behaviors is the pain face or pain mask. The forehead is wrinkled, eyebrows furrowed, eyes slightly closed with the corners down turned, cheeks drawn and tight, jaw slightly clenched, and a drawn-out wince or grimace. This mask can be continual or happen mainly with postural changes from standing to sitting to lying down. This look says, "I'm in pain, constipated, or angry."

Indeed, the families and friends of pain sufferers will often say, "He always looks angry." As a result, people may avoid the pain sufferer, especially children and strangers because of the vaguely threatening quality of the pain mask. This can interfere with your getting the support you want or using socialization to distract yourself from pain. On the other hand, because it can tell people to stay away, it is an effective way of letting you climb into your cave and hole up if that is what you want.

Occasionally a patient at one of our clinics will have some type of intervention, usually an injection that provides her complete pain relief for a time. She smiles, laughs, and is obviously happy and relieved to be pain free. But sometimes, except for her smile, the rest of her face doesn't know she is happy and pain free. The pain mask has become such a habit that it has settled into her wrinkled forehead, furrowed eyebrows, slightly closed eyes, and tight and drawn cheeks even when she is pain free or nearly so. In a few instances, we have asked patients to look in the mirror and slowly arrange the rest of their face to match their smile. It can be very revealing, and sometimes even humorous, to let patients see how much their facial expressions are controlled by pain or the residual of it.

WHAT ARE POSTURAL PAIN BEHAVIORS?

There are other postural or static pain behaviors. When people hurt, they often tighten up their bodies, especially in or near the area that hurts. Frequently, we observe chronic, severe tension in the neck and shoulders, often identified by raised shoulders, and a rigid torso. This can be so extreme that patients hardly move their neck and head from side to side independent of their torso. Rather, they seem to move everything above the waist as a single unit. This is an example of "anticipatory bracing" and is perfectly natural when you have pain. You hurt and you anticipate hurting worse. Your body tenses up in anticipation of hurting worse and out of stress and fear. When you are stressed or anxious, your nervous system becomes more aroused and one aspect of that arousal is increased muscle tension, most severe in the painful area.

Another postural pain behavior is referred to as "guarding." You may hold or carry an injured body part in an artificial, distorted manner that seems to prevent worse pain. People with shoulder, arm, or hand injuries may hold or cradle their arms or hands in an awkward, distorted manner that feels more comfortable, but that in the end increases pain. Someone with neck pain that radiates down an arm may position that arm in a limp manner making the arm appear as if it were injured or paralyzed. Someone with back pain, especially with pain that radiates down a leg, may twist his back, pelvis, or leg in an unnatural position that seems more comfortable but that also increases pain over time.

In addition to standing postures, sitting postures are almost always distorted to one degree or another with various types and locations of musculoskeletal pain, particularly spinal, abdominal, or leg pain. A patient may enter the office and sit down mainly on his left side, leaning his left elbow on the arm support, with his left buttock supporting most of his weight and his right leg slightly raised and extended. His body is screaming, "My back and right leg are killing me, do something," although that may not be the intention.

Some patients with back pain do not sit in a chair with a 90-degree angle formed by the shoulders, buttocks, and knees. They may have their buttocks pushed forward in the chair so that they are more nearly forming a straight line with their shoulders, stomach, and knees, as if they were halfway between lying and standing. This usually happens when bent legs cause more pain or sitting up straight hurts worse.

WHAT ARE MOVEMENT-RELATED PAIN BEHAVIORS?

Pain behaviors affect not only standing and sitting postures but walking or other movements, also. A common behavior with certain types of spine, hip, or leg pain is to over or under-rotate your hips when you walk, as well as limping or dragging your leg. With upper extremity or hand pain, you may carry your hands or arms in a distorted manner when you walk to prevent increases in pain.

A patient of mine, June, demonstrated one of the most severe pain behaviors I have ever seen. She had neuropathic pain in her left hand and arm that was also sympathetically mediated, and diagnosed as Reflex Sympathetic Dystrophy. Her left hand was clawed. Her wrist was rotated so her palm faced upward with her thumb against the palm of her hand, and her fingers were partially curled over the thumb. When standing or walking, her right hand held her left hand in this position. When sitting, she rested her "claw" on her stomach, again cradled in the other hand. Of course, the claw prevented her from using the hand at all, effectively making her severely disabled.

When I discussed this issue with her physician in a team conference, he indicated that the claw was not an actual contraction but a preference or habit. Frankly, I did not believe him. At her next appointment, I asked her if she could straighten out her hand. She did so, quickly and easily. I think she noticed my surprise. She commented that the clawed position felt more comfortable for her and that other people were less likely to bump into her terribly sensitive arm if they saw her hand clawed. The problem was that by not using her hand, it would wither and weaken. In this event, she really would lose permanent function of her hand. Thus, the most critical aspect of our treatment became increasing the use of her hand and eliminating the anticipatory claw.

How Can Pain Behaviors Increase Pain?

Anticipatory bracing, guarding, and un-natural movement changes all result in a host of problems that increase pain. With asymmetrical muscle recruitment there is a difference in how each side of the body is working, whether it is right and left arms, or right and left legs, or opposite shoulders, or even opposite sides of the spine. The more injured side tends to be favored, leading to overcompensation by the non-injured, stronger side and escalating weakness of the injured side.

We can revisit an earlier example and gain fresh insight. If you have pain in your left side low back and left leg, the right side back and right leg may eventually compensate for the left. In biofeedback, we may document much more muscle activity or tension in the right side back, even more so with standing or walking. Over several years, this right side muscle activity may increase as the left side back and leg become weaker and the muscles atrophy. Weak muscles atrophy, i.e., they contract or shrink. In the low back, this contraction of the injured left side weak muscles can actually pull the left side hip and pelvic girdle up toward your spine. To better understand this process, you can do this yourself.

To illustrate, stand up straight now if you can and place your hands on your hips with your feet flat on the floor. Lean to your right and raise your left hip up a couple inches so your left hand and elbow is now higher than your right. You may notice that your left heel comes off the floor and you have most of your weight on your right leg. Over time, your pelvic girdle and hips can become almost locked in this position, making your left side progressively weaker since it is bearing less weight. As time passes, it is very likely that your right hip or knee will begin to hurt, and may eventually become damaged from overcompensation. Okay, you can sit back down now. Thanks for helping.

The above is also a perfect example of why chronic pain is more affected than acute pain by factors other than the original tissue damage. Favoring one leg over the other because of leg or back injury does not significantly increase pain for many months or years until muscles begin to weaken and the body makes adjustments. Bracing, guarding, and overcompensation are also behaviors that are part of the suffering aspect of the pain experience. They open additional pain gates in the low back while increasing the excitatory activity of A-Delta and C-pain fibers.

Another complicating factor with bracing, guarding, and movement-based problems like limping is referred to as poor muscle recovery. Whether caused by injury or overcompensation, tight, constricted muscles do not perform as well as healthy ones. Muscles perform work by contracting or shortening from their relaxed resting state (baseline) and then returning to a relaxed state after activity is over. A healthy muscle returns to the same amount of muscle tension after activity, as it possessed before. An unhealthy muscle does not always relax completely. It maintains a little more muscle tension after an activity. In isolation, this is not a big problem, but with repeated episodes of activity over the course of a day, the residual muscle tension following activity produces gradually escalating muscle tension and pain.

Figure 10 demonstrates how repetitive, incomplete muscle recovery can increase muscle tension throughout a day. In this figure, a person in pain has tightened a muscle numerous times during a day. You can see that the difference between the peaks and valleys is getting smaller throughout the day. This occurs because the person is maintaining additional, residual tension in the muscle with each contraction. This increases the average muscle tension over the course of a day. It is highly likely this person will have increased pain as a typical day progresses.

Figure 10: Escalation in Daily Muscle Tension for a Person in Pain

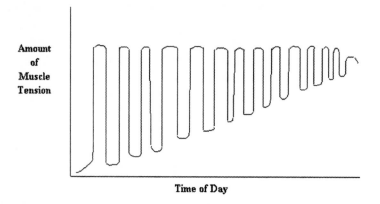

HOW DOES A BIOFEEDBACK THERAPIST DECREASE PAIN BY CHANGING POSTURAL AND MOVEMENT-BASED PAIN BEHAVIORS?

It is nearly impossible for most chronic pain sufferers to make healthy changes in anticipatory bracing, guarding, muscle recovery, or body movement distortions on their own. However, this is the career work of a Certified Biofeedback Therapist trained in chronic pain. Most modern biofeedback equipment uses sensors placed on the body at strategic points to receive physiological information and transfer the signal to the biofeedback equipment with a mini-processor that analyzes the information. The biofeedback unit is usually connected to a personal computer that displays the information on a video monitor for both visual and auditory feedback.

With chronic pain sufferers, the biofeedback therapist places electromyographic (EMG) sensors around the site of injury. These sensors are connected to the biofeedback equipment that uses computer graphics to display muscle tension, contraction, or spasming. During the initial consultation, the therapist will usually assess muscle activity so that you will be able to see on the computer monitor your own anticipatory bracing, guarding, spasming, weakness, etc. Further, your therapist will assess muscle activity across different postures and movements, e.g., sitting, standing, moving, and using your arms. This allows you to see your body's compensatory strategies or poor muscle recovery. Of equal importance, you will learn from your experience in biofeedback sessions that as your postural and movement-based muscle tension changes to a more normal level, your pain almost invariably decreases.

This experience with biofeedback can be almost magical for many pain patients. In an individual biofeedback session, pain may decrease from 70/100 to 30/100. Headaches may go away. Even neuropathic pain can be significantly improved. These changes are not automatically permanent. When you leave the office, all the old habits and pain may return, but you will have seen the correlation or bridge between voluntary behaviors and pain. You will have learned that there are subtle bodily changes you can make to cross the bridge, and reach a place of reduced pain and increased function.

Over the course of twelve to sixteen sessions, the biofeedback therapist will teach you hundreds of strategies for maintaining healthy neuromuscular posture and movement. This is the most powerful method for experiencing how a great deal of your pain is caused not just by tissue damage but by other factors, too. You are given practice exercises to use at home and will feel encouraged and hopeful.

At our clinic, whenever possible, patients will have back-to-back sessions with me and the biofeedback therapist. I have met with many patients after their initial session of neuromuscular re-education and heard them express frustration that they had not been referred for biofeedback training earlier. Recently, a woman commented that she thought biofeedback training should be a requirement for all patients with chronic pain. While that may not be true, biofeedback training is one of the most powerful weapons in the arsenal of pain treatments.

Talking About Pain

Another common pain behavior is talking about pain. When you are sick or hurting, you tend to talk about it. The pain is new and interesting. It may mean something that is worth talking about. Hopefully, the caring people in your life have rallied around you, at least a little, to provide loving support and comfort as appropriate. Pain is extremely stressful, and most of us like to talk about the stressful things in our lives.

Talking about pain and pain-related events causes you to think about your pain more than you would otherwise. If you are withdrawn and inactive, you may not have much else to discuss other than pain-related topics. Unfortunately, we learned that thinking about pain opens pain gates by decreasing inhibitory pain impulses and chemicals sent to the dorsal horn of the spinal cord. This means that at the most primitive biochemical level, talking about pain makes it worse.

In future chapters we will discuss at length the devastation that chronic pain brings into the lives of those afflicted. For now, we can say that the profound life changes wrought by chronic pain and the misery of the experience combine to make it a natural topic of conversation. Initially, this will be interesting to your family and friends. As your condition drags on, however, and you do not make the expected recovery, the topic becomes stale or worse. Family and friends don't know what to say or do. They feel increasingly helpless. The chronic nature of your condition, and your unhappy response to it, may begin to make them less interested in your company, or at least your conversation. The more you talk about your pain, the more your family and friends are confronted with it, and feel expected to say or do something about it.

Most of the patients with whom I work will tell me that they have learned not to talk much about their pain. They have learned that "people don't really want to hear about it anyway so I hardly ever talk about my pain." Then I bring their most important support person into a session and that person says, "We are constantly talking about his pain," much to my patient's surprise and indignation. Sometimes people talk about their pain more than they realize. Sometimes support people define *talking about pain* differently than patients do.

From a patient's perspective, talking about pain is saying something like, "God, my back is killing me today." From a support person's perspective, however, it may include the moans, groans, and grunts you make when sitting down or standing up. They may believe that you are talking about your pain when you discuss doctors' appointments or treatments you are receiving.

For support people, talking about pain may include talking about unemployment, physical limitations, Social Security, worker's compensation, or finances. It may seem that you are talking about pain, or at least your medical condition any time you discuss a myriad of things related to your lack of complete recovery. To a support person, it may feel like you are talking about your pain any time you verbally express anything that makes them have to deal with the reality of your medical condition.

It is important that you be able to talk about the practical, real-world consequences of your condition, so that you and your family can plan and adjust. However, it is not helpful to actually talk about your pain or to wince, moan, groan, grunt or otherwise communicate that you hurt. There are several reasons why it is best to change these behaviors to the extent that you can.

When people have a limb amputated, the world rallies around them for a time. After their condition stabilizes and they complete rehabilitation, the fact that they are missing a limb slowly becomes a familiar part of them. That's just the way they are. Patients stop talking about what it is like to be an amputee and support people stop asking questions. Their disability becomes a less worthy topic of conversation.

A chronically painful, physically limiting medical condition needs to become as integrated into the person in pain as a missing limb is to an amputee. People in pain and their family and friends need to stop treating the condition as an acute, short-term illness and begin integrating it into their lives and their relationships. Then, both patients and support people will talk about it less. This allows the person in pain to begin normalizing the experience, in the same way that an amputee must normalize the loss of a limb or a diabetic the need to inject insulin regularly. In each of these situations, people must stop putting their lives on hold until the pain or disability goes away. They need to make their condition feel as normal to themselves and others as possible.

A related pain behavior is how people talk about their pain. I pay close attention to the language people use in describing their pain. If they refer to their condition as being sick or ill, they have clearly not accepted the chronicity of their painful condition and they are probably soliciting their support system to continue rallying around them. Chronic pain is not a sickness or a progressive disease and it should not be described as such. It is a terrible, stressful condition, as is losing a limb, but neither are diseases.

Most people with chronic pain can provide an exhaustive list of things they used to be able to do but *can't* anymore. Over time, they may discuss in excruciating detail all of the things that they *can't do* anymore. However, many of these activities are possible for them to perform with sufficient motivation.

Jill was a patient who told me that she was too weak to lift more than ten pounds anymore. She got very angry when I asked her if she could throw my twenty-pound computer through the window if that was the only way she could get out of the burning, flaming room. Eventually, she agreed that she could, and got even angrier when I summarized the discussion by saying, "So you can lift more than ten pounds."

In Jill's mind, she was telling the truth, even though she lifted her twelve-pound walker out of the car routinely. What she meant was that it caused her pain to lift ten pounds or more and that she could only do it infrequently. My point was that she usually *chose* not to lift ten or more pounds because the costs were greater than the benefits—a logical, healthy decision, but not one based upon can or can't as much as based on choice.

It has been my experience that the more people in pain resist this notion of choice, the less willing they are to commit to self-responsibility for their own pain. The more they cling to the bosom of victimization, the less likely they are to help themselves. The language of can and can't destroys your motivation and promotes a not so stoic, passive suffering, rather than the determination to combat your pain with all the tools possible. Pay close attention to what you tell yourself you can't do, and, whenever possible, acknowledge that not doing an activity is usually a choice, probably a healthy one, but still a choice. You will feel a greater sense of control, and more a master of your own fate.

Some people in pain demonstrate a lack of integration in the way they refer to their injured body parts. When someone says, "The leg doesn't support me," or "The arm won't let me write anymore," they are rejecting or disowning parts of their body. They are psychically splitting. They are saying, in effect, "There is the old, healthy part of me and this new damaged part that really isn't me; it's an alien that I must rid myself of to feel whole again." This is incredibly unhealthy thinking and virtually guarantees poor coping behavior. Every time you use this type of language, you reinforce dis-integration and lack of wholeness. You are not incorporating your changing abilities into your self-perception. You will tend to obsess about how your life would be but for the rejected parts of your damaged body, or will be once your damaged parts stop being damaged. Either way, you are more likely to keep your life on hold.

MISCELLANEOUS PAIN BEHAVIORS

Even more subtle examples of pain behavior are attending doctors' appointments, going for diagnostic testing, and taking medications. You would not engage in these behaviors if you did not have pain. Pain behaviors can also involve how patients deal with doctors and medical appointments. "Doctor shopping" is an example of a pain behavior in which a patient goes from one doctor to the next, each time hoping for a brand new treatment, surgery, or cure. Often, these patients carry tales of perceived mistreatment by previous doctors, or at the very least, the belief that the doctor had given up on them, or had nothing else to offer. Sometimes, the patient's mission becomes finding that one doctor who will provide a definitive diagnosis or special level of understanding.

As we discussed previously, doctor shoppers usually switch providers near the end of the Exploring stage of treatment. They are the medical equivalent of serial daters who cannot commit to a long-term relationship. I consult to a few dozen competent, board certified pain physicians in Southern California. They read the same journals, attend the same conferences, and mostly provide similar services. If a patient has been miserably unhappy with the first three pain doctors, the fourth one is likely to lose his luster quickly, too.

HOW TO MINIMIZE PAIN BEHAVIORS

Minimizing pain behaviors is often referred to as "acting *as if*." You can act as if you did not have pain; as if you were more functional; as if you were not so depressed. The more you surrender to your pain with the myriad of possible pain behaviors, the stronger you communicate to yourself that you are damaged goods. This leads us to another problem with talking about pain.

It is a fact that people talk about short-term, immediate crises more than long-term concerns. You will talk more about not being able to pay this month's rent than you will the size of your retirement, at least until the rent is paid. The more you talk about how much you hurt, the more you convince yourself that your pain is a short-term crisis and not an integral part of an emerging you. Worse still, you attribute your talking about your pain to the fact that it is short term, as do the people around you. This is partly why they feel frustrated when the pain does not end. They were rallying around you with the expectation that their efforts would be short lived. When the pain does not go away, they do not want to maintain that level of support. And you may need to stop acting as though your pain will be gone tomorrow if they will just hang in there for now.

Occasionally, I work with a person in pain whose family or friends do not want him to stop talking about pain or minimize pain behaviors. They are described as so caring and supportive that they would be upset if they knew that the person was hiding or minimizing his pain. This is an incredibly unhealthy pattern of interaction. You become a walking advertisement for pain and medical problems. You are unwittingly being encouraged to define yourself as a pain sufferer not as a spouse, parent, employee, or volunteer. Remember, the more time you spend talking about your pain, the more you reinforce it, the more you open pain gates, and the more you hurt.

You must realize that many pain behaviors you absolutely cannot or should not change, or eliminate. If it feels like you are stepping on broken glass or sharp rocks every time your right foot hits the ground, there are limits to how normally you will ever be able to walk. If you are taking medication, you will need to attend an occasional doctor's appointment. Throughout your day, you may experience and engage in many healthy behaviors, which are a partial function of the fact that you hurt, e.g., using a heating pad or ice. Your task is not to avoid all pain behaviors, but to minimize them as much as is healthy.

In Chapter 6, we acknowledged that the longer you have pain, the more your doctor is interested in estimating where your pain lies on the pain sensation-suffering continuum. This should and will affect the treatment decisions he makes. The easiest and most obvious source of information available to your doctor is your pain behavior within the pain clinic and during your formal appointments.

There are pain behaviors that will push your doctor's perception of your place on the continuum toward the suffering end. Examples include: sobbing at every appointment; constantly being angry or conflicting with staff; screaming when you receive injections; showing up without an appointment; refusing to stand because it "hurts too much," but then walking to your car; always describing your pain as at least a 90/100; and frequently asking for pain shots. True or not, fair or not, these behavioral patterns tend to be interpreted as increased suffering and poor coping, not necessarily increased pain sensation.

Begin to notice the presence and frequency of your pain behaviors in all areas of your life. Ask family or friends how often you engage in these behaviors. Work on making some changes in your pain behaviors and periodically ask your support people how you are doing. You can integrate strategies for improving pain behaviors into your Personal Pain Paradigm. You will be surprised at how much this reduces your pain and suffering.

I know that decreasing pain behaviors can ease some of my pain and suffering

Insight—I understand the various unhealthy pain behaviors.
Commitment—I am committed to decreasing my pain behaviors.
Action—I will begin monitoring my pain behaviors and enlist the aid of my support system.
Now—Today I will change one unhealthy pain behavior, and that behavior is:

_____
_____
_____.

10

How to Pace Yourself and Set Healthy Limits

Effectively pacing yourself and setting limits with your activities are the hallmarks of good self-management, and a critical element in your Personal Pain Paradigm. They require a scientific approach to pain through the development of a pain record in your TAAP journal. For a one-to two-week period, you should regularly write down all your activities and your pain level. For this period, document your activities in as much detail as you can. How long did you sit, stand, walk, lie down, use the computer, or do light chores? You should also track your pain level every one to four hours on a scale of 0-100.

For these first two weeks, the pain record is your teacher. You will get the answers to several important questions. What times of the day do you tend to hurt worse? Which activities increase your pain? Which decrease your pain? How much of the day do you spend resting or lying down? How much do you spend on your feet? People who take the time to produce a pain record are often surprised with the results. The pain record allows you to plan healthy changes that are specific to your unique condition.

WHY IS SETTING LIMITS IMPORTANT?

Setting limits with your activity is at the core of the successful management of your chronic pain. Limit setting is the antithesis of the philosophy of "no pain, no gain" that is seen so often with acute pain treatments and sports medicine. An argument against limit setting could be made because increases in pain caused by simple daily activity are not harbingers of increased injury. Standing on your feet a little too long or sitting at the computer too long may increase pain, but will not actually injure you more.

Perhaps your task might be to just tough it out using all the mental gymnastics you can. This is wrong for several reasons. First, every time you overdo, you hurt worse, which makes you suffer more than is necessary. You do not have to suffer more. There is no benefit to your suffering more. Remember, pain and suffering is bad, period.

Second, each time you overdo, you teach yourself inaccurately that activity is painful, and that you *can't* do certain activities, or at least not without terrible pain. The more you reinforce this notion, the more restricted your activities become and the worse your quality of life. This makes you feel even more disabled.

Third, each time you overdo, you do not just increase pain for a little while, but may have worse pain for hours or days afterward. A pattern of repeatedly poor limit setting can cause continually increased pain and decreased activity, during which time you may get weaker, more dysfunctional, and probably more frustrated.

Give yourself permission to ask for help with tasks that are grossly beyond healthy limits. Some activities inevitably increase pain. Vacuuming, mopping, carrying laundry, and grocery shopping are perfect examples of high pain tasks. There may be twenty other light chores combined that do not cause as much pain as any one of the above four. You may have less pain throughout the day if you do the twenty other chores and ask someone else to either take over these high pain tasks or help you do them.

I can appreciate that in the real world you cannot always avoid doing things that exceed healthy limits. However, there are times when it seems like you "have to" and times when you simply "want to" for other reasons. For instance, you might decide to spend eight hours at Disneyland with out-of-town relatives knowing it will "light up" your pain like the Fourth of July. In these situations, you should still minimize overdoing as much as possible.

With grocery shopping, ask for assistance. Accept help from the bag boy with your groceries. Wait for your strapping son to carry in the bag of dog food or help you put away heavy items on high shelves. You will not always get the help, but at least you can ask for it. This does not make you dependent. On the contrary, it allows you to save energy and manage pain for other perhaps more important tasks.

I hope it is clear that the consequences of overdoing far outweigh the benefits. The consequences can be extreme or long-term even if they do not cause increased tissue damage. Activities should be performed to tolerance, where tolerance is defined as that level of an activity you can perform before your pain increases by 10 on a scale of 0-100. As a rule, do not do things that reliably and significantly increase your pain, no matter how tough you are, because eventually your coping ability will break down and your overall level of functioning will decrease.

WHY IS IT IMPORTANT TO PACE YOURSELF THROUGHOUT THE DAY?

Pacing your activities is the corollary of setting good limits. If you do not perform any given activity past the point where it increases your pain by 10 of 100, or by 1 of 10, then you will be changing your activities frequently during a typical day. Healthy pacing requires that you repeatedly change your activities throughout the day to maintain a relatively level amount of baseline pain with few severe pain peaks.

In Chapter 3, we discussed how chronic pain always fluctuates, and we described the two most common pain patterns. Unipolar pain patterns generally have increasing pain as a day progresses. Bipolar patterns have high pain in the morning, lower pain around midday, and higher pain again toward the end of the day. With both of these patterns, pain that increases toward the end of the day is often caused by poor pacing and limit setting, which can induce poor muscle recovery and overcompensation. Good pacing requires a scientific approach to a day's activity. You need to be proactive and change your activity before your pain increases much.

The standard pacing mantra in the field of pain management is to "move your muscles and change your thoughts." True pacing is not merely varying what you are doing, but what you are thinking. You are essentially refreshing yourself dozens of times throughout the day. This is especially helpful when you are anxious, frustrated, or angry and spending a lot of time obsessing about the things that are making you miserable. Changing your posture and activity is a great way to shake off darkly negative thoughts and regroup.

HOW TO VARY YOUR ACTIVITIES TO DECREASE PAIN

The four basic postures that use different muscle groups are standing, sitting, lying down, and walking. Good pacing requires that you vary these positions, continually rotating them throughout the day based on the goal of avoiding a pain increase of 1 of 10 or 10 of 100 from any activity. For example, you might stand while doing things with your hands for fifteen minutes, before you notice that your pain is starting to increase. You can sit down and feel comfortable for maybe thirty minutes before noticing that your pain is starting to increase. Then, perhaps you walk and move around for about twenty minutes before your pain begins to worsen. Then you might lie down or recline for forty-five minutes before your pain starts to increase.

This cycle of four activities took a total of 110 minutes. Since we want you to change activities before your pain increases, you might subtract five minutes from each activity. This would create a ninety-minute cycle: ten minutes standing, twenty-five minutes sitting, fifteen minutes walking, and forty minutes reclining. You could repeat this about ten times in a typical, sixteen-hour waking day.

You probably do not have any idea how much or for how long you can perform each of these basic activities before your pain begins to increase. This is another instance where your TAAP journal is valuable. If you complete a pain record for a week or two, it will include a log of your regular activity for a week. You will notice that you vary your activities naturally and you can get a sense of how long you perform each activity.

After completing your pain record, spend a few days vigorously committed to changing activities and positions before your pain goes up by 10 of 100. These days should be days in which you are not gainfully working or have too many heavy chores. Document this trial period in your TAAP journal also. At the end of the trial, look at your TAAP journal and it will tell you about how long on average you can spend doing any one activity before the hounds descend. This schedule should form the basis for and length of your baseline activity cycle. Remember to subtract a few minutes from each activity like we did in the example above to ensure that you change activities before pain increases.

The more severe your pain and physical limitations, the more frequently you will change activities. The worse your pain condition, the less time you will probably spend standing or moving, and the more time you will spend lying down or sitting. To improve your quality of life and ability to complete daily tasks, your long-term goal is to increase time spent standing, walking, or moving around while decreasing time spent lying down or sitting.

Lying down is a unique situation. Since your overall goal is to be more active with less pain, you do not want to lie down throughout the day more than you absolutely must to manage your pain and cycle healthily through activities. You might plan to set the lying down periods at about 30 minutes initially and see how your body and your cycle work with 30 minutes of complete rest. You may find that you need to change this length of time either up or down.

Give your body one to four weeks to adjust to the baseline cycle schedule. This is defined as the maximal activity you can perform that prevents pain from increasing by 10 of 100 for a given activity. As your body adjusts to the cycle schedule, you can slowly begin to increase the amount of time you spend standing or moving and decrease the amount of time you spend sitting or lying down. If you need to be able to sit for long periods to perform much of your work, then you may want to focus on extending your sitting time. The rule of thumb is not to increase your time in an activity more than 10 percent, per cycle, per week. If you were able to move around comfortably for thirty minutes continuously per cycle, you would not increase your time by more than three minutes per cycle in a given week.

The above regimen might seem logical and based on common sense, but how in the world do you keep track of all these times? For a while, you will need to use a timer, a stopwatch, or an alarm clock. This is a great deal of work and very inconvenient. But, I almost guarantee that if you follow the steps from creating your baseline pain record to establishing a healthy activity cycle, you will learn something incredible. You will learn that you overdo multiple times throughout the day. You will also learn that you increase your pain unnecessarily on a regular and frequent basis. You are repeatedly being caught up in a task or project, and exceeding your limits without realizing it, until it is too late.

PATTERNS OF ACTIVITY ASSOCIATED WITH POOR PACING AND LIMIT SETTING

The effects of poor pacing without a healthy activity cycle are reflected in the most common patterns of activity throughout a typical pain day. The first pattern is seen in Figure 11. We see high activity during the early part of the day that quickly decreases to low activity for the rest of the day. In this figure, someone is very active for as long as he can tolerate it, and before he crashes until the next morning.

This activity graph is a companion to the unipolar pain pattern we described earlier. If you have low pain in the morning that escalates as the day progresses, you are likely to have higher activity in the morning with decreasing activity as the day progresses.

Figure 11: Unipolar Daily Activity Level with Chronic Pain

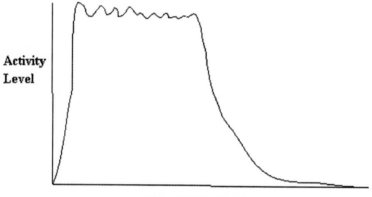

Time During the Day

The severely decreased activity "crash" in Figure 11 may come at Noon, 3:00 p.m. or 6:00 p.m. Usually a patient in pain will say that she is inactive later in the day because she has to be; she simply cannot keep going all day. This may be true but only because she does such a poor job of limit setting and pacing earlier in the day. She may comment that she accomplishes more in a day, if she crams it all together and then rests. This is simply not true.

The second common daily activity pattern is seen in Figure 12. Here we note high activity in the morning, less activity early to mid afternoon, and increased activity again later in the afternoon before a crash again in late evening. This activity pattern is also usually the result of poor pacing and limit setting early in the day, which produces a crash in late morning or early afternoon. After a few hours of rest, this person is either able to regroup comfortably for a few hours of repeat overdoing, or feels compelled to do so because a child or spouse has come home with a new set of demands.

Figure 12: Bipolar Daily Activity Level with Chronic Pain

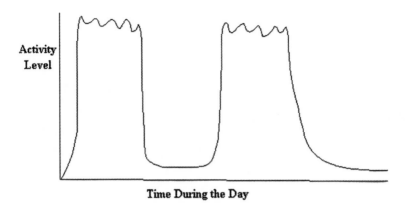

Time During the Day

Figure 13 shows a person who is setting healthy limits and pacing well using all four postural activities including lying down. We can see this person repeatedly cycling through all four basic postures during a day.

Figure 13: Healthy Pacing in Daily Activity Level with Chronic Pain

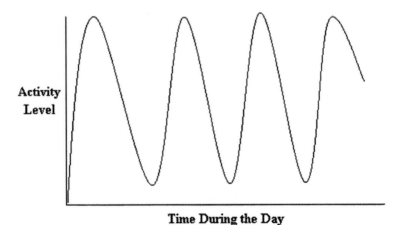

Time During the Day

If we compare Figures 11, 12, and 13, you will notice that the average level of activity is higher the more frequent and shorter are the rest periods. This means that with frequent rest periods, the total amount of resting is less because you need less rest. Why? Because you are not escalating your pain through overdoing, and then trying to manage that increased pain. If you tell me that you have to lie down for three hours in the middle of the day, I will believe you. But, I will know that it is because you are pacing and limit setting very poorly throughout the morning.

How to Structure a Pain-Filled Day to Get the Most Done

Your Personal Pain Paradigm includes a highly structured approach to daily activity though the use of your TAAP journal, pacing, and limit setting. Structure is the soulmate of chronic pain. Spontaneity and lack of structure are pain's evil mistress. They seduce you with, "I do what I can and rest when I have to," which usually means, "I overdo repeatedly and then crash miserably."

Structure and organization allow you to keep going throughout the day, to progress through both pleasurable and productive activities. Structure also helps you feel less victimized and helpless. Structure says, "I still have some control over my life." Structure is not quite as sexy as spontaneity, but it is the best possible life partner.

Many people in pain lose the fabric of their life's structure, the foundation of their daily activity. Most people with severe chronic pain are not employed full time, even if they were before their pain began. Gainful employment structures your day more than you realize until you are unemployed. If you work from 9:00 a.m. to 5:00 p.m., your early mornings are spent preparing for work, and your early evenings are spent decompressing and performing necessary domestic chores. This means that about fourteen of sixteen waking hours are accounted for from Monday through Friday. The weekends are organized around fun, social engagements, and all the chores you did not have time for during the workweek.

If you were not employed outside the home when your pain problem began, you probably still carved out a busy, structured day with domestic chores, errands, shopping, appointments, or children's activities to complete before dinner and bedtime activities. You too may have had fourteen of sixteen waking hours accounted for, just Sunday through Saturday, instead of Monday through Friday (a domestic goddess doesn't get the weekends off).

Chronic pain can bring both employed and stay-at-home, busy lifestyles to a screeching halt. Your inability to perform your usual tasks or maintain your usual routine may leave you feeling adrift, rudderless, and completely disconnected, in some primitive way, to the rest of the world. As previously suggested, many people in pain will say, "I do what I can, when I can." Sometimes this means "I do very little and only when I get around to it."

The compelling force in a busy person's life is the second part of Newton's First Law of Motion: "A body in motion tends to stay in motion," or rephrased, "A busy person tends to stay busy." The first part of Newton's First Law is that "a body at rest tends to stay at rest." With people, this is referred to as the couch potato phenomenon. Combining these two body principles we learn that it is much easier to stay busy than to get busy. When you have an unstructured and inactive life, habits and inertia are working against you, not for you. That grinding, head down, "I'll just keep putting one foot in front of the other until the weekend comes" mentality is lacking.

An old phrase that I have always liked, perhaps because I think it applies to me, is, "If you want a job done, give it to a busy person." That person will not procrastinate. She will jump on it and give it only as much time as is necessary before moving on to the next job in the long list. Without structure or inertia on your side, every task seems larger than life. Every task requires that you create the inertia of movement and the structure necessary for the task. Without structure, people regress into obsessing about the most unimportant things, or worse, truly dark things over which they have no control. They turn small tasks into big ones.

Gravitate toward people, places, and things that promote and encourage healthy pacing and limit setting. Organize your life around situations that make it easy to be good to yourself. For example, if you want to be faithful to your spouse, among other things, don't spend a lot of time drunk in singles bars with your single friends who happen to hate your spouse. Similarly, if you want to manage your pain effectively, don't volunteer to cook Thanksgiving dinner at your house for twenty of your relatives. You should be watching football that day. And since you're not hanging out in singles bars anymore, maybe your spouse will cook the dinner. Just a thought.

The point is that there are situations in which you know that you will not set good limits or pace yourself well. It is supremely dishonest to experience one of those situations to the fullest and then be surprised when you wake up in terrible pain, or with a stranger. It is also unacceptable in this situation to expect that your pain physician should consider this an emergency and save you from the consequences of your choice or poor judgment.

I am not saying that you should never overdo, never give yourself permission to throw caution to the winds. There are times when you will decide and probably should decide to work or play too hard. But these situations should be relatively rare, saved for special occasions, and with you fully accepting of the consequences.

Healthy pacing and limit setting are the keys to a better life with pain

Insight—I understand the strategies for pacing and limit setting.
Commitment—I am committed to setting limits and pacing myself better.
Action—I will log my baseline activity pattern and practice my activity cycles.
Now—Today I will be more mindful of activity-based increases in pain.

11

How to Set Goals and Achieve Them in Spite of Pain

Goal setting is an extremely effective way to establish healthy structure in your life. Perhaps more than any other comment I hear from people in pain is this statement, "I used to have goals; now I just feel like I'm drifting." In the context of rehabilitation for chronic pain, you can set goals for physical, social, pleasurable, or productive activity. The goals should be realistic, measurable, and achievable through actual behaviors that have an endpoint. "Getting rid of my pain," may not be a realistic goal. "I want to be less stressed" is not readily measurable either. "I want to be stronger" is a realistic, measurable goal, but we need to identify the behaviors that help you achieve greater strength.

Goal setting is a mechanism for healthy change. Goals anchor your Personal Pain Paradigm into daily activities. Good goals represent healthy changes that you want to make in your life. They identify the direction in which you want to proceed. You can translate the life changes you want into goals by asking yourself the same types of questions I ask my patients. If you want to be happier, what would that look like? What are the most important things you would be doing differently if you were happier? Most patients will still identify very general changes. "I would be able to do more stuff," or, "I would have my old life back."

The following five basic criteria for establishing goals are:

- *G*ood

- *O*bjective

- *A*ttainable

- *L*earning and

• *S*ustainable.

WHY SETTING GOOD GOALS IS IMPORTANT

A good goal is one that is healthy, both mentally and physically. It is reasonable and consistent with common sense. It is not an idle wish, like, "I think I'll learn Greek this year." It is something that you have really thought about and is important to you. You want to feel enthused about your goal. You want it to motivate you and encourage you through the process. It should be constructive—something that will make you a better person.

WHY YOUR GOALS SHOULD BE OBJECTIVE

An objective goal is one that is concrete and tangible. There should be no doubt when you have achieved the goal. It is measurable and characterized by behavior, which is really the only objective measure of human experience. "I want to lose twenty pounds" is measurable and concrete but not something that you can do by force of will. It requires multiple, specific behaviors which are themselves objective.

In fact, Matt was a patient who actually did want to lose twenty pounds, but when we analyzed the reason, it was because he wanted to lose his bulging stomach and make it definitively smaller than his chest. He assumed that losing about twenty pounds was the way to do that. However, if we focused on the objective goal of getting his stomach to a size smaller than his chest, weight loss would become only one of several strategies to accomplish that goal.

He could also do resistance training three times a week to increase his chest size along with several abdominal exercises to flatten his stomach. Unfortunately, I am reminded here of the cartoon that shows two women exercising on the floor of their gym. One of them smiles at the other and says, "Before I started doing stomach crunches, I had a big, soft belly. Now I have a big, hard belly." Weight loss is important, too.

Making goals objective often requires translating them into behavior. You might think, "I want to be happier." "I want to be more like my old self." "I want to feel some purpose again." These are great things to want, but they must be translated into objective goals. I ask my patients, "What would it look like if you were happier? What would you be doing that would make you happy?" At this point, we can begin developing a list of behaviors that would lead to or represent happiness. These behaviors would become your objective goals.

We have already identified several healthy goals in this book. General goals include decreased pain, increased function, and the creation of your Personal Pain Paradigm. We have also discussed goals that are more specific. It is healthy to maintain your TAAP journal, minimize pain behaviors, and gradually increase physical activity. You should determine your stage of medical treatment, and then decide how you want your treatment to proceed. It is important to establish baseline pain and activity levels within effective pacing and limit setting. Each of these goals is represented by specific and measurable behaviors.

WHY HEALTHY GOALS MUST BE ATTAINABLE

Good, objective goals must be attainable. This can be the most difficult aspect of goal setting for people with chronic pain. Let's look at Fred, for example. He stated his treatment goals very simply to me, "I want to be able to work and exercise as I did before I got hurt. When one doctor runs out of ideas for curing me, I go to the next. I won't give up."

I suggested to Fred that after fifteen years and eight spine surgeries, he was never going to be able to do all the things he could do before his injury. I expressed the belief that he needed to accept that fact and get the most out of life that he could. He did not return after our initial appointment. Fred's goal was unattainable and unhealthy. I was unwilling to collude in his fantasy. He chose to find another doctor who would.

WHY LIFE GOALS SHOULD PROMOTE GROWTH AND LEARNING

Setting healthy goals within your Personal Pain Paradigm promotes learning. You should learn something from accomplishing a goal. Certainly, attaining the goal itself is enough reward, but you should gain some insight into a healthy strategy, a characteristic, or some other aspect of yourself. Herein often lies the real, hidden benefit of goal setting and accomplishment—the fact that you can learn something for life that you can add to your hierarchy of coping strategies.

It is important to record in your TAAP journal what you are learning as you go along. Note which things worked and which didn't work. What you learn from working toward a goal helps you incorporate specific goals into the general plan of your life, and you gain true wisdom.

WHY GOALS SHOULD BE SUSTAINABLE

Finally, goals should be sustainable. They should include only behaviors that you can maintain for the length of time you have set aside for attaining that goal. You might establish the goal of exercising three times a week for the next week and subsequent weeks. However, exercising daily for the rest of your life may not be sustainable. It is important that your goal not be so effortful and dramatic that it exhausts you and makes you realize you could not sustain it long term. Like life, managing pain effectively is a marathon, not a sprint. You want to readjust your lifestyle on a long-term basis, so you must have goals you can maintain.

TIMEFRAMES FOR GOALS

There are three types of goals: short, medium, and long-term. Short-term goals are accomplished in a day or a week, such as, "Today, I will stretch my back three times." Or, "I will do a breathing exercise every day this week."

Medium-term goals are completed in a week to a couple of months. These include projects with multiple necessary behaviors. You might decide that over the summer you will clean the house, and get rid of all the junk. Each week you will take one room, clean it, and put the junk in the garage. The final two weeks of the summer, you will go through the junk, throw away whatever you cannot use, and then have a garage sale to get rid of the remaining junk. Medium-term goals must be translated into short-term goals or they will never be done. So you might say, "I will spend twelve hours cleaning the kitchen this week, and I'll divide that chore up into six, two-hour segments with breaks every thirty minutes." Another example would be to say, "Today, I will clean out the junk drawers between noon and five o'clock, pacing myself along the way."

Long-term goals may take from a few months to many years. Jack, for example, was planning his daughter's wedding over an eight-month timeframe. He wanted to be able to walk her down the aisle and dance with her without using his walker. In consultation with his physical therapist, we established a month-by-month graduated plan of rehabilitation, breaking down each month into weeks, and each week into daily tasks. He did walk his daughter down the aisle and got the first dance with her. There wasn't a dry eye in the house. Kudos to Jack.

In Chapter 10, we noted that a structured lifestyle is the foundation for good pain management. Goal setting and goal attainment are strategies for developing structure when pain seems to be a barrier to structure at every turn. "I do what I can" seems like common sense, but it leads to doing very little. "I do what I plan" leads to the structure that creates a satisfying life, in spite of some pain.

Chronic pain can devastate almost every aspect of your life. You can watch yourself disintegrate from a Type A, go-getter, worker bee who never sits still, to a passive lump, a shell of your former self. The road back lies along the path of goal setting, planning, and carving out the life you want—maybe not the one you had before, but a whole lot better than the one you have now.

Setting realistic goals and working toward them is almost impossible until you become honest with yourself and accept the chronicity of your condition. Then you can show the necessary courage to stop waiting to feel better before you move forward. Even then, it takes tremendous independence to create a new life that incorporates pain. You need to be flexibly creative when establishing goals and planning how to overcome obstacles. You will need to initiate behaviors for the goals you set and persevere with a sense of relentless purpose. Thus, the pain resistant personality and seven life choices are crystallized in setting and achieving goals.

The GOALS strategy for structure can guide my activities and sense of purpose

Insight—I understand how to set goals that are Good, Objective, Attainable, Learning, and Sustainable.

Commitment—I am committed to structuring my life activities through goal setting.

Action—I will establish short, medium, and long-term goals.

Now—Today, I will accomplish one small goal that I might not have otherwise, and that goal is:_____

_____.

12

How to Exercise Even if You Suffer from Pain

If you have chronic pain, physical exercise is probably the single most important thing you can do to lessen your pain and enhance your quality of life. It is also the hardest thing to do. This may prove that God has a sarcastic side, or that he picks on the meek before he lets them inherit the earth. I have discussed the importance of physical exercise with every pain class I have ever led. At least one person will look at me as if I'm nuts while thinking, "It took every ounce of strength and willpower I had to make it into this clinic today, and you want me to exercise? Where's my Danskin® leotard and who let him graduate?"

THE TROUBLE WITH TRADITIONAL REHABILITATION EXERCISE

The majority of patients in pain will say that their pain increases throughout the day and especially with activity. The vast majority will say that they cannot perform physical exercise because it hurts too much. They have learned to associate significant physical activity with pain, either from overdoing it on their own or in physical therapy.

As your body gets weaker from lack of exercise, the association between increased activity and increased pain may be reinforced, as it takes less and less activity to increase pain. Life activities may constrict as you feel trapped by your withering body. Traditional approaches to physical exercise will fail. You need exercise strategies that are specific to your chronic pain.

Once you experience pain, all the treatments you receive are directed toward your painful area. Why? Because insurance companies pay physicians and therapists to work on pathological processes to recover normal health. Put another way, the traditional medicine industry helps patients go from sick to well, not from well to even healthier. Every medicine, therapy, injection, or surgery is directed toward your aching back, neck, arms, head, stomach, etc. No one is interested in the parts of you that do not hurt, or those parts that are healthy. Even you are becoming increasingly more focused on the parts that hurt. We all know "the squeaky wheel gets the grease."

In the meantime, those healthier parts of you are not getting much attention and may not be getting any exercise, either. Therefore, they are getting weaker and less healthy, every single day. Inactivity is strongly associated with increased muscle pain around the original site of your pain or injury. We also know that weak muscles can hurt independent of injury or tissue damage.

It is estimated that the human body loses about 1-3 percent of muscle tone for each day of bed rest. In a month or two of bed rest, you become a jellyfish. The less you exercise and the more inactive you are, the more likely it is that you will hurt worse as your muscles become weaker. This is independent of any change in your original pain problem. The bottom line is that weak muscles hurt more if they are not exercised.

For example, let's say that you strained your back and developed a small (3 mm) bulging disc. You may take several days off work to rest. This allows your back to heal somewhat, but it also makes your back weaker. If you continue to rest or to be inactive for weeks or months, your back muscles will continue to get weaker, which means that they will get shorter and feel tighter. It is very likely that eventually you will feel increased pain, even if your disc problem or lumbar strain improves. Why? Because weak muscles hurt.

Many people in pain who don't exercise are not lying in bed 24/7, but they do spend a significant amount of time inactive or "vegging out." Certainly, the area around their injury is getting weaker, but so is the rest of their body. In fact, the rest of the body can eventually become as weak as the injured parts. As this happens, the rest of the body begins to hurt, often in a pattern that spreads out from the original painful body part. In many cases, people end up with almost total body pain due to their inactivity and globally weakened muscles, not because of an underlying disease process. Remember, weak muscles hurt.

WHY EXERCISE SHOULD EMPHASIZE THE LEAST INJURED BODY PARTS

Since weak muscles hurt and people with chronic pain end up with varying degrees of weak muscles, a rehabilitation program that focuses mainly on the original, injured area is almost doomed to fail. The rest of the body passively waits for the original painful area to get stronger before its turn comes around. However, the rest of the body never gets a turn, because the painful part may never get stronger. The uninjured body parts just keep waiting and devolving; becoming the ever-weakening chain that is only as strong as the weakest link. The first priority of a physical rehabilitation program for chronic pain should be to get the rest of the body as strong as possible to help pull up the weakest link.

Although exercising the least painful body parts probably makes sense to you, insurance companies will not pay for this rehabilitation strategy, and most certainly medical treatment will not emphasize this. Physicians and insurance companies must focus almost entirely on damaged or diseased areas of the body. You must exercise the rest of your body on your own, as one more element in your Personal Pain Paradigm. Medical providers cannot, in any meaningful way, assist you in this process.

The physical therapy model of increasing strength, endurance, and flexibility (range of motion) is a good one and consistent with general health measures. In the world of basic exercise and health maintenance, strategies for increasing these measures of health are usually referred to loosely as resistance training, cardiovascular exercise, and stretching.

THE IMPORTANCE OF AEROBIC EXERCISE FOR CHRONIC PAIN

Let's begin with endurance or cardiovascular exercise. Endurance or stamina is improved mainly through aerobic exercise, which can allow you to maintain 70 percent or less of your maximum heart rate for at least twenty to thirty minutes. With aerobic exercise, you get enough oxygen to support an activity over time. Running and swimming can be aerobic exercises. Weight lifting and sprinting are examples of anaerobic exercises that can only be performed briefly or for a few repetitions before the body fatigues from oxygen debt.

Aerobic exercises provide incredible short-term benefits as they speed up your metabolism, improve digestion, and promote well-being by producing endorphins and enkephalins, nature's natural painkillers. Long-term benefits include lowering your resting heart rate, strengthening your immune system, and increasing serotonin, a neurotransmitter that levels out negative emotion.

Meaningful aerobic exercise is impossible to perform when it uses your painful, damaged body parts too much. This is one of the common problems with physical therapy. You may start with heat, ultrasound, and massage, and then graduate to gentle stretching or strengthening. Then, your therapist may talk about doing some "cardio" and put you on the treadmill. Being able to walk is critical for independence and ease of life activities, but, if your pain is orthopedic, or is exacerbated by impacting, weight-bearing exercise, you may never be able to use walking as a truly effective aerobic exercise.

Keep in mind what your aerobic exercise goals are if you have chronic pain. First, you want to produce endorphins and enkephalins, which are nature's natural painkillers. These chemicals actually increase your pain tolerance.

How Does Aerobic Exercise Increase Pain Tolerance?

Nociceptive pain tolerance is defined as the amount of pain that you actually experience from a given painful stimulus. Pain tolerance research has often been conducted using the cold pressor test. Subjects immerse their hands in a bucket of ice water that is a constant temperature, about 34 degrees. Your pain reaction is measured based on verbal report, nervous system arousal, etc. If person A demonstrates in every way that he is experiencing more pain than person B does, we would say that person A has a lower pain tolerance than person B. From the same physical stimulus, he experienced a higher level of pain. Clearly, this is an imprecise attempt to measure a completely subjective experience, and yet we acknowledge that people have varying pain tolerances. In this context, pain tolerance is not defined by how much pain you can stand, but rather, how much pain you actually experience from a given painful stimulus.

Numerous factors affect pain tolerance including genetics, physiology, psychology, motivation, distraction, etc. You know that thoughts, feelings, and behaviors affect pain experience and tolerance, but you also know that various cells and chemicals that are present in your body can either increase or decrease your pain sensation.

Excitatory and inhibitory processes in nerve cells (neurons) can increase or decrease pain. Neurons communicate with each other through chemicals called neurotransmitters, which are found in the tiny cleft between adjacent neurons, where the end of one neuron (axon terminal) almost touches the beginning of another (dendrite). These neurotransmitter chemicals can have an excitatory or inhibitory affect on pain signals and either increase or decrease pain. Most important to pain perception are the neurotransmitters called endorphins, enkephalins, serotonin, gaba, and norepinephrine.

Receptor sites for endorphins and enkephalins are concentrated in the dorsal horn of the spinal cord and work on a lock and key model to decrease pain. These particular neurotransmitters travel to the same receptor sites as do prescription narcotics to decrease pain exactly as do narcotics—by locking up the receptor site so it cannot send pain messages to the brain. We have also referred to this as closing the pain gate. Long story short, the more endorphins and enkephalins you have in your body, the less pain you will experience from a given painful stimulus, i.e., the higher your pain tolerance.

So how do you get more of these natural painkillers into your body? You get them through aerobic exercise, mainly. Vigorous cardiovascular exercise activates many body systems including the brain's production of natural opiates. Evolutionarily, aerobic exercise was associated with either running toward food to kill it or running away from beasts that considered us food. Either way, we needed to be more impervious to pain and discomfort, hence the rapid influx of endorphins, enkephalins, and other neurotransmitters that inhibit pain. However, to produce these chemicals in large amounts, the aerobic exercise must be vigorous. From our perspective, you need to minimize how much you use your damaged body parts and maximize how much you use your healthier body parts in order to exercise vigorously enough to produce healthy amounts of endorphins and enkephalins, which in turn, increase your pain tolerance.

Aerobic exercise also causes the brain to produce other neurotransmitters, serotonin being the most important for pain. Serotonin is a nonspecific neurotransmitter that has a wide range of effects including improving pain, mood, and sleep. Though not a natural opiate, serotonin has been demonstrated to have an analgesic or pain relieving effect. Decreased serotonin levels are associated with lower pain tolerance and depression.

Increased pain tolerance is not the only reason aerobic exercise is important for patients with chronic pain. Aerobics burn more calories than any other form of exercise, which promotes weight loss. Additionally, aerobic exercise increases metabolism for twenty-four to forty-eight hours after the exercise. This means that your body continues to burn more calories at rest for one to two days after you have exercised. Since most patients with chronic pain gain weight and this weight often increases their pain, weight loss can be a critical component of a Personal Pain Paradigm.

How to Select a Pain-Free Aerobic Exercise

There are hundreds of additional benefits from aerobic exercise independent of chronic pain. Your task is simply to get your heart rate up through exercise for a designated period of time. So, how do you minimize the use of your damaged body parts? For most people in pain, especially those with musculoskeletal problems, selecting an exercise begins by learning the hierarchy of the four basic types of musculoskeletal exercises. They are categorized by a combination of the proportion of your weight that you must support and the amount of impact or jarring on your joints. From easiest to hardest, these exercises are labeled: 1) non-impact, non-weight bearing; 2) non-impact, weight bearing; 3) non-weight bearing, impact; and 4) weight-bearing, impact exercises.

For most people in pain, non-weight bearing, non-impact exercises are the easiest aerobic exercises. These exercises include activities like pool (aqua) exercise or recumbent bike, i.e., a type of stationary bicycle where you lie virtually flat on your back with your legs parallel to the ground. You do not have to support your own weight when you are on your back or in chest-deep water. Bicycling is non-impact because your feet stay in contact with the pedals and this prevents jarring. Water provides enough resistance that even walking in the water is non-jarring. Almost anyone with any type of pain problem can exercise in the water without increasing pain or risking further injury. You can simply walk back and forth in the shallow end. You can do deep-water walking or jogging using a flotation device. You can join exercise classes offered at many pools, sometimes referred to as Hinges and Twinges. Or you can swim in a modified way.

The least demanding swimming stroke is on your back using the elementary backstroke. This requires that you put your hands all the way out to the side, so that your body looks like a cross and then you pull your arms down to the side while simultaneously doing a frog kick. If you cannot use your legs, you can put a flotation device between your legs and let them go limp. As you get better at this stroke, you can begin reaching your arms over your head to get a longer pull. You could ask someone at the pool to show you the elementary backstroke. The next easiest stroke is probably the sidestroke, followed by the breaststroke.

Perhaps the best way to introduce you to the benefits of water exercise is through aqua therapy, a type of physical therapy performed in the water. Many patients and doctors do not know that water therapy exists or is helpful. For many chronic pain patients, it is the only type of exercise that is sufficiently aerobic for pain reduction. Since you may not be very vigorous in the water until your body is much healthier, it is important that the water is very warm so you are not chilled. Therapeutically heated pools are 89 to 93 degrees Fahrenheit. This is almost ten degrees warmer than a typical recreational or lap swimming pool.

Water is the great equalizer and lowest common denominator; virtually everyone can exercise in the water. You are capable of water exercise unless you have an open wound, are receiving oxygen 24/7, or are otherwise profoundly disabled. You may have legitimate barriers to water exercise such as finances or lack of transportation. In this event, you may want to explore other exercises, perhaps with the direction of your physician.

The second easiest type of aerobic exercise is weight bearing, non-impact exercise. It is not jarring, but requires you to bear some or all of your weight. Examples include an upright stationary bike, hand bike, stair climber, rowing machine, elliptical trainer, cross-country ski machine, stair stepper, cardio glide, etc. If you are able to do any of these exercises reasonably comfortably, you may want to start with them rather than the recumbent bike or pool. You are always better off having one of these machines in your home, which takes the trip to the gym out of your list of excuses for not exercising. Certain types of "power" yoga can be cardiovascular as well as strengthening, i.e., they are non-impact, and vary between weight bearing and non-weight bearing.

The next type of exercise would be a non-weight bearing, impacting exercise. However, there really are no examples of this type of exercise since any exercise that is impacting is also weight bearing. Underwater boxing could be a theoretical example of this type of exercise.

The fourth and most difficult type of aerobic exercise is weight bearing, impact exercise. Examples include walking, jogging, boxing, and formal step aerobics. With these exercises, you are bearing most or all of your weight. Because your feet or hands do not remain in contact with something at all times, the exercise is jarring. It affects your body. Most people, including physicians and physical therapists, think of walking as an easy, entry-level cardiac exercise. This is absolutely not true for patients with musculoskeletal pain.

Of the four basic types of aerobic, total-body exercise, walking is included in the most difficult category. It compels you to bear all of your weight, and the pounding forces that are generated on your heels and the balls of your feet are extreme—up to thousands of pounds per square inch. Walking can aggravate or "light up" your pain regardless of whether your pain is in the arms, legs, neck and shoulders, low or mid-back, abdomen, or originates from headaches. You may never be able to walk with sufficient speed to produce aerobic benefits. This does not mean that you should omit walking as an exercise. It's just that walking is usually not sufficiently aerobic.

How to Pace Yourself So Aerobic Exercise Does Not Increase Pain

Your task is straightforward, if not easy. Select one of the four classes of exercise and begin doing one or more on a regular basis, multiple times each week, for the rest of your life. Over time, from weeks to years, you may graduate to a more difficult class of exercise. Now that you have chosen a potentially pain-free exercise, let's turn our attention to how you should exercise when you do have pain.

The key to all physical exercise with chronic pain is to exercise within the model of good pacing and defined limits. This means you should not significantly increase your pain, during or after the exercise. You learned that "no pain, no gain" may be a good model for world-class athletes trying to make a living, but it is extremely unhealthy for those with chronic pain. When you overdo with exercise, you reinforce the idea that trying to increase your activity is painful. When you overdo, you will eventually take a break from the activity or exercise as you wait for your body to return to its baseline pain level. This interrupts your schedule and results in your losing many of your hard fought gains. If you overdo even 10-20 percent of your exercise sessions, you may never be able to progress.

You need to determine how much of your selected exercise you can perform before your pain goes up by 1 of 10 or by 10 of a 100. If your exercise is in the pool, you will need to experiment with different types of movements and length of time spent in the water. You may start with slowly walking around in shallow water or doing deep-water walking.

If your exercise is with a machine, you will need to start on a slow speed for a short period. You can then increase your exercise time if you are able. Your goal is to reach a minimum of thirty minutes. Regardless of which exercise you choose, you are better off focusing your initial efforts on increasing the time up to thirty minutes and only after that goal has been reached should you increase the speed or intensity.

Once you have established a baseline type and amount of exercise that does not increase your pain by even 1 of 10 or 10 of 100, you are ready to set up a schedule. We would suggest that you begin with about 50 percent of your baseline amount. If your exercise was walking in chest deep water and you can do that for twenty minutes before your pain begins increasing, then you should begin exercising for ten minutes daily.

Only this exercise approach allows you to exercise every day. Even on your higher pain days, you can do the exercise without further risk of increasing your pain. If you tried to exercise the full twenty minutes, on high pain days, your pain would probably increase further. The cornerstone of this approach is that it allows you to exercise every day. You need to exercise nearly every day to improve chronic pain. Mild, daily exercise increases benefits and decreases risks.

Some types of exercise for various groups of people do not significantly increase pain at the time but do afterwards. In this event, you would need to moderate your exercise even further to prevent increasing pain after exercise. The key is to exercise daily, and thus eliminate the "no pain, no gain" mantra from your vocabulary. You may not be aware that a small amount of delayed onset muscle soreness is fairly common within twenty-four to forty-eight hours after exercising.

For years, experts have talked about exercising moderately, three to four times per week, for twenty to thirty minutes each time. This is one of many great lies foisted on us by the medical and health establishments. This was never enough exercise and the experts knew it. They just believed that if they told us how much we really needed to exercise, we would get discouraged and stay on the couch. They figured that any amount of exercise was better than none.

Physical therapy is often set up this way, on a Monday-Wednesday-Friday type of schedule. The assumption is that you will need to have a rest day in-between exercising to allow your body to recover, heal, and grow stronger. The problem is that with chronic pain, if your body needs a day off to recover, you have probably overdone it and are hurting worse. This reinforces the belief that increased activity is painful and you will probably still hurt worse even after the day of rest. If you adhere to that schedule, it is just a matter of time before you break down and have to stop exercising.

Ideally, you will get into a rhythm of mild, gentle, daily exercise for a couple weeks and then begin increasing time spent exercising by no more than 10 percent per week, ever. Once you are up to thirty minutes, you can slowly increase the intensity or speed of the exercise. This is not an exercise program that you will do until you feel better, and then stop. This is a lifelong component of your Personal Pain Paradigm designed to help you feel better and improve conditioning.

Aerobic exercise applies only to your non-injured, healthier parts. The other two aspects of musculoskeletal health are flexibility and strength. They both apply to your injured and non-injured parts. For most painful conditions, you will want to focus more on strengthening the non-injured parts and more on stretching the injured parts—both strength and flexibility are important. Interestingly, like pain relief and improved function, in some respects strength and flexibility are the same thing.

STRATEGIES FOR FLEXIBILITY, STRETCHING AND STRENGTHENING WITH CHRONIC PAIN

Flexibility is increased in the body trunk and limbs by stretching and lengthening the muscles and connective tissue, e.g., fascia, tendons, and ligaments. When muscles are underused, they begin to atrophy or waste away as they contract and become shorter. Muscle strength is largely determined by how much a muscle can contract from its resting state. A muscle that is short and already contracted cannot contract much more and thus is weak and prone to injury. A long, supple muscle can contract greatly from a resting state.

Stretching Exercises for Chronic Pain Management

The primary strategy for improving flexibility is stretching. These exercises should be performed by gently holding a stretch for twenty to thirty seconds, neither bouncing nor letting something force you to stretch farther. You should begin by gently stretching the pain-free, non-injured parts and then only after you are warmed up, even more gently stretch the injured, painful parts. If it hurts, don't do it. You will find it easier to stretch in warm water, in a heated room, or when wearing warm clothes. You can get stretching exercise examples from a physical therapist, books, or articles about your particular pain problem. Yoga and Pilates are very popular exercises for conditioning, since they include both stretching and strengthening.

Massage Therapy for Chronic Pain Management

Massage is another wonderful strategy for increasing flexibility and promoting general health. Massage is probably the most underutilized of all the possible strategies for pain management. Almost every patient who experiences massage even in a limited way in physical therapy will sing its praises. A good massage can elongate and relax angry, sore muscles and connective tissue in places you did not even know were angry and sore. It also eliminates toxins and stimulates the release of neurotransmitters and other healthy chemicals. Some patients will reject massage as being too expensive, an average of $50.00 to $75.00 for an hour. A half-hour massage is cheaper and you may be able to get even more reduced rates by signing up with a massage school where massage therapists in training are learning their craft.

A typical massage schedule consists of weekly to monthly visits. If you are making co-payments for muscle relaxants, anti-anxiety medications, anti-depressants, or anti-inflammatories, a regular massage may reduce or eliminate these costs. Bodywork can dramatically improve your quality of life and that of the people around you. It can be the most cost effective thing you do. You may not be able to afford regular massage, but it may be that massage needs to become a specific priority, just as your self-management needs to become a general priority for you.

Strengthening Exercises for Chronic Pain Management

Strengthening exercises are usually applied to the non-injured areas, but should also include the muscles and connective tissues associated with the painful area. Resistance training is the gold standard for strengthening. The idea is that your muscles must resist or move weight, whether your own or an artificial weight, and those muscles will get stronger by adapting to a higher workload. In addition to Yoga and Pilates, formal weight lifting and using therapeutic bands are examples of resistance training. As was true for stretching, you should begin by focusing more on training the non-painful areas, and only after at least a month of resistance training, begin to incorporate the more painful areas. If it hurts, don't do it.

The best approach is to employ high repetitions (twelve to fifteen) using light weights. Do not do as much as you can. Do not "max out" or exercise to failure. If you are doing a chest-pressing exercise, begin with a weight you can press fifteen times with relative ease. Do fifteen repetitions, three times with rest and then move to another exercise. You can do four to six exercises, and then stop for the day. Never increase your weights by more than 10 percent per week.

HOW TO INTEGRATE EXERCISE OF PAINFUL AND PAIN-FREE BODY PARTS

You can do strengthening exercises six days per week if you alternate muscle groups or do upper body one day and lower body the next. With strength training, you gain more benefit by allowing the exercised muscles twenty-four to forty-eight hours rest as long as you are strengthening some other part in-between. It can be helpful to stretch before doing resistance training and so you may combine stretching and strength training daily.

By developing a program of resistance training, aerobic exercise, and stretching, you are exercising more than three to four times per week. In fact, the rule of thumb is to approach fourteen times per week. You might do your aerobic exercise daily in the morning and stretching or resistance training in the evening, or vice versa. If you are able to stick to this type of schedule for a few months and feel confident with it, for time reasons, you may vary your activity. For instance, if you chose lap swimming as your aerobic exercise, it is considered high repetition resistance training, due to the strength required to propel yourself through the water. You might decide to taper formal resistance training to three or four times per week. If you work full or part time, you might modify this schedule and alternate your aerobic and resistance training days. You need to be practical and fit exercise into the demands of your life, but I would strongly suggest that you work up to the fourteen times per week model of exercise, and maintain it for at least a month.

In Chapter 8, I stated that people in pain apply the same hierarchy of strategies to pain that they have applied to every other life situation. People who exercised regularly before they developed pain tend to exercise regularly after they have pain, if they are taught how to exercise properly. People who did not exercise regularly before they had pain are unlikely to begin exercising after they have pain even if they learn proper techniques. This latter group has even more reasons not to exercise now.

For the vast majority of people in pain, barriers to non-painful exercise eventually degenerate into excuses. Here are a few I have heard over the years:

• The water frizzes my hair and makes it turn green

• I don't want to be seen in a bathing suit

• Riding a bike is so boring

- I hate going to the gym

- I have no one to exercise with

- I've never really been an exerciser.

Almost inevitably, these excuses really mean, "I'm not motivated enough to help myself feel better." If that is true for you, and if you know right now that you are capable but unwilling to begin even the simplest, non-painful exercise regimen, you may want to stop reading. Then acknowledge that you will never feel much better, and have another injection or pill. Meanwhile, keep telling your doctors and family, "I would do anything to feel better."

If you have chronic pain and do not exercise, you are severely limiting how much benefit you can receive from anything the doctors do for you. Integrating a regular exercise regimen into your daily routine is probably the single most important thing you can do to have less pain and be able to function better. The greatest tragedy of my professional life has been watching thousands of patients who would like to feel better refuse to exercise and handicap themselves and their doctors for the rest of their misery-filled lives. I truly hope you will not be one of the tragedies. Now, it's up to you.

Exercising is the most important strategy in the self-management of chronic pain

Insight—I can exercise daily without increasing my pain.

Commitment—I am committed to improving my strength, flexibility, and endurance.

Action—I will choose, plan, and initiate a program of resistance, stretching, and aerobic exercise.

Now—Right now, I will choose the healthiest aerobic exercise for me, and that exercise is: _____

_____

_____.

13

How to Blend Healthy Daily Activity and Movement into Your Schedule

Physical activity during a typical day affects everyone with chronic pain differently. Some people are most comfortable lying down, some sitting, some standing, and some moving around. These are the four basic body postures or mechanics we discussed in Chapter 9. You should vary your activities between these four postures on a regular basis throughout the day. But even within these four posture groups, you can better manage your activity to accomplish more during a typical day. For this chapter, our model will describe orthopedic and neuromuscular pain, though the concepts apply to almost every pain condition.

WHY SOME DAILY CHORES HURT MORE THAN OTHERS

As an introduction, a lesson in body mechanics will be helpful. As you sit there, let your hands hang down by your sides and feel how easy and natural it is. Now, keep your arms rigidly straight and raise them until your hands are shoulder height in front of you. Hold them there while slowly counting to sixty, and notice the tension and fatigue in your arms and shoulders as your arms resist gravity. After awhile, your arms and shoulders will become uncomfortable and would be painful if you held your arms out like that for a few minutes. Now drop your hands so they hang down by your sides again.

Imagine that you have a ten-pound weight in each hand as they hang down by your sides. If you kept your arms straight and slowly raised them to shoulder height, you would notice that the ten-pound weights felt as if they were heavier the closer your hands came to shoulder height, and held further away from your body. If you then slowly brought the outstretched weights into your chest at shoulder height, they would feel progressively lighter until they were pressed against your chest. If you then dropped the weights down to your sides and then let your hands hang again by your sides, the weights would feel lighter still. What's going on here?

The mechanical concept that matters here is force of rotation or torque. The weight of an object multiplied by the horizontal distance the object travels from its axis equals the foot-pounds of torque. In the above example, the shoulder joint is the axis. In other words, the rotational force (torque) comes both from the amount of weight you are lifting (ten pounds) and the horizontal distance that weight is from the shoulder (about twenty-four inches with arms fully extended).

You can increase foot-pounds of torque by moving a heavier weight or moving the weight further away from you. From a musculoskeletal perspective, the more torque required, the more strain on the joint involved and all ancillary muscles and joints. Lifting a weight out and up places strain not only on your shoulders and arms, but also on your neck, low back, and knees, etc. These joints have to resist or counteract the force of rotation. As the weight of the object or the traveled distance increases, so does the strain on those other joints. In Figure 14, you can see the geometry of your body's lifting torque and strain.

Figure 14: The Relationship between Torque and Strain or Effort

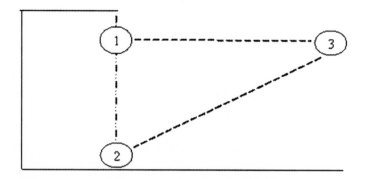

The dotted line between points 1 and 2 in Figure 14 represents the vertical centerline of your body. This line proceeds from your heels upward through your legs, hips, and spine to the top of your head. If you are lifting an object from point 2 to point 1, there is no rotational force (torque) at all, so the object will feel only as heavy as it really is. But, if you lift an object from point 2 to point 3, your shoulder joints have to create tremendous rotational force and other involved muscles and joints have to support that force.

When you hold a weight out at point 3, your body is naturally pulled forward in the direction of the weight. To hold your body steady and not let it be pulled forward, you must resist being pulled forward using all the related ancillary muscles and joints, e.g., low back, neck, and knees. This can require intense effort and place severe strain on your shoulders and most of the rest of your body. Your body treats an object lifted to or held at point 3 as if it were much heavier than an object lifted to or held at point 1.

Intuitively, you already understand this process as it relates to lifting and holding things. If you try to lift a suitcase that is two feet in front of you by bending deeply at the waist, it will impose severe torque on your spine, shoulders, and arms. Instinctively you will try to minimize torque, effort, and strain by moving closer to the suitcase before lifting it, if possible. This explains why you might be able to carry luggage onto a plane rather easily, and then you struggle to lift it up and hold it out, while placing it into the overhead compartment. This principle is the foundation for the familiar maxim, "lift with your legs, not with your back."

The heavier the object you are lifting or the further out you hold the object from the centerline of your body, the more torque is required. But, increased torque also increases the effort and strain on all the ancillary body parts. When you have lifted an object to hold it shoulder level with your arms fully extended, it feels as if it were many times heavier than when you hold that same object down by your side. In other words, an object held shoulder high at arms length challenges your legs, spine, and shoulders, a factor of many times more than an object held at your sides.

Our bodies are remarkably strong and capable of supporting and handling heavy loads when they are close to our bodies and create little torque. Larger, stronger people may be able to carry bags of dog food on their shoulders or pressed against their chests that weigh 80-100 pounds. Yet, we are poorly adapted to move even lightweight objects a distance away from our bodies.

You know that you may be able to lift and carry fifty-pound suitcases in each hand straight down at your sides, but hold maybe only ten or fifteen pounds at shoulder height straight out in front of you. Most people would find it easier, less tiring, and less painful to lift and support fifty-pound weights carried at their sides, where there is no torque, than to lift and support ten-pound weights on their outstretched hands, where there is tremendous torque. Very few people could ever hold even thirty pounds straight out in front of them for more than a few seconds.

How much effort or strain does holding a piece of paper place on your neuro-muscular and orthopedic systems? You might think that because it weighs less than an ounce, there is minimal effort or torque involved. Except, how about the weight of your arm itself? From the body mechanics exercise that began this chapter, you demonstrated that your empty hand held out-stretched in front was too heavy to hold out for long without discomfort. Your arm from shoulder to finger tips weighs between about five and fifteen pounds although the torque and strain required to lift and hold it out makes it feel many times heavier. Given the weight of your arm and hand, holding a piece of paper at arm's length will challenge your musculoskeletal system as if you were supporting 15-100 pounds near your body's centerline. With this information, we are ready to take a fresh look at the physical demands of various domestic activities throughout a typical day.

The Physical Demands of Vacuuming Chores

Let's look at vacuuming. For most people with chronic pain, vacuuming hurts. Why? Imagine you are vacuuming and you have just pushed the vacuum head all the way forward. Your back is bent slightly forward, your arm is completely extended, the wand is three to four feet forward of your arm, and there is a one to five pound head at the end of the wand. The torque involved in this task is extraordinary.

We said that with your arm fully extended, an object in your hand felt as if it were many times heavier than one at your side, in terms of the musculoskeletal strain needed to support it. An object held out further than your hand (the wand) strains your musculoskeletal system much more, and the further out from your hand an object is held, the heavier it feels (the head). A vacuum cleaner wand and head that weighs five to ten pounds total can place extreme strain on your musculoskeletal system and feel as if you are pushing and pulling well over a hundred pounds. Moreover, bending at the waist, even in isolation, produces severe torque on the structures associated with the spine. No wonder vacuuming hurts!

The Physical Demands of Laundry Chores

How about laundry? The ten-pound basket of laundry you carry in front of you with your arms nearly extended can strain your musculoskeletal system as if it weighed many times as much. After the laundry finishes the washing cycle, you have to lean forward (producing torque), extend your arms into the machine (more torque), and pull the wet, heavy clothing away from the side wall (more torque). Then you must lift the clothes out of the washer before placing them in the dryer. You have to repeat this several times. You can easily be challenging your musculoskeletal system as if you were manipulating hundreds of pounds of laundry. The mechanics of pulling laundry out of the dryer are similar, although you are lifting a little less weight since the clothes are dry. Further, the process of folding clothes and putting them away requires hundreds of repeated episodes of extending your arms out in front with a small weight at the end of them.

The Physical Demands of Food Preparation Chores

What about cooking? The same process and mechanics apply. Standing and reaching for the plates, silverware, food, pots, pans, glasses, etc. requires significant musculoskeletal strain as many as hundreds of times over a period of twenty to sixty minutes. Some of the actions produce surprising amounts of torque and strain on ancillary body parts. Removing that one-gallon carton of milk on the top shelf of the fridge requires enormous levels of torque with severe stress on your body. The saucepan held out by the handle with a ten-pound combination of water and pan at the end of the handle may feel as if it were many times heavier. Worse still, some of these activities require holding your arms out for a length of time.

Light Chores May Increase Chronic Pain

In sum, any household activity that requires extending your arms produces much more strain on your musculoskeletal system than would the same activity without your arms extended. This strain is caused by the combination of foot-pounds of torque (weight multiplied by distance) and ancillary body parts being compelled to resist the forward pull created by extending your arms. The strain on your body is even greater with an object in your hands and greater still the heavier the object or the further it extends. If you bend at the waist or stoop, the strain of an activity with arms extended is maximized further. In this way, seemingly light chores can actually be hidden, heavy labor that dramatically increases chronic pain.

How to Decrease Pain While Doing Daily Chores

Successfully managing most chronic pain problems requires the effective management of physical energy and work. You need to become more mindful of how you conduct your daily activities. In this context, we refer to the green, yellow, and red zones of activity performed while sitting, standing upright, or moving.

The Green Activity Zone

The green or go zone represents activity performed with your hands at your sides or immediately in front of you, about waist high, with your hands almost touching your stomach. This is maximally energy conserving and minimizes the effort and torque needed to perform an action.

The Yellow Activity Zone

The yellow or caution zone represents activity performed with your hands out in front enough that your elbows and shoulders line up with your hips or are slightly in front of your hips. Your hands will be about six inches in front of you and may be a few inches above or below your waist. If you have neuropathic or musculoskeletal pain, performing activities in the yellow zone is about as much as you should challenge yourself on a frequent basis.

The Red Activity Zone

The red or stop zone is activity performed with hands out in front far enough that you appear to be reaching and can feel tension in your shoulders. Red zone activities include those performed more than a few inches above or below your waist. It is best to perform these types of actions as infrequently as possible. With a red zone activity, the further you reach or the more weight you are moving, the greater the likelihood of increased pain. The more frequently you perform red zone activities, the greater the likelihood of increased pain.

For most people in pain, it is also best to minimize bending, stooping, or twisting as much as possible. These activities increase torque and musculoskeletal strain severely and can increase or cause pain. These actions are even riskier when they are done quickly or when your body is not warmed up. Notice as you go through a day how often you engage in these activities.

How to Organize Your Home to Decrease Your Pain

At this point, you can begin to look at the ergonomics of your home with a fresh perspective. Spend an hour with pen and paper walking through your home and see how it is set up for the physical demands of simple chores. Your reference frame can be: hands at waist level, up front, and in close are good and place you in the green zone. Hands high or low, behind you, or not close in front are bad and place you in the red zone.

Reorganize Kitchen Items

Begin in the kitchen. Do you keep the plates you use three times a day up high at eye level while the spices you use once a year are on the counter at waist level? Are the heavy pots that you frequently use kept at about knee or foot level? Do you use the top shelf of the fridge at eye level for heavy milk and juice, and the waist high levels for light vegetables, cheese, or yogurt? Each of these examples would be increasing your musculoskeletal stress and probably your pain.

Give yourself permission to be creative. Think about what items you actually use daily and do your best to keep them in the green zone, even if that means placing them where they do not seem to belong. The builders of your home did not plan for you to have chronic pain and they may have been taller or shorter than you. Some of your cupboards may extend flush with the counter below them, but some may be indented forward 6-18 inches, which compels you to reach or even bend forward to access them.

If you routinely use only a few dishes, cups, or pots in a typical day, you might keep them out of the cupboard or put them in a special place at waist level. Perhaps a few plates could go in the junk drawer you never use. Maybe some pots could be hung on a hook inside the pantry. If you use dish soap three times a day, why should it be kept under the sink? Perhaps you could put frequently used items in movable shelves on the counter. Do you keep a footstool nearby to help you reach for those items that are a little too high? Do you have the financial resources to redesign certain aspects of your kitchen to make it more pain friendly?

Reorganize Bathroom Items

Now go into the bathrooms. How are they arranged? Do you keep items that you use every day above or below the counters and not on them? Where do you keep the towels or toilet paper? In the shower, where are the soap, washcloths, razors, and shampoo located? Would it help to attach liquid dispensers to the wall or hang a basket below the showerhead? How often do your bathrooms compel you to stoop or reach?

Reorganize Bedroom Items

Look in the bedrooms. Where do you keep frequently used clothes, shoes, socks, and underwear? Could you move things around to spare yourself some unnecessary reaching, lifting, bending, or stooping? Would it help to elevate your bed? Could you get your shoes off the floor by hanging a shoe carrier on the door?

Reorganize Main Living Areas

Check out the family room, den, and living room. Notice how these rooms are organized. Where are the items you use every day? How are the couches and chairs arranged? Could you change anything to make your life easier? If you spend most of your time in these rooms, small changes can yield big results.

You can become more mindful of the thousands of times every day that you reach, lift, or perform an activity that is outside the green zone. Based upon what we have learned in this chapter, let's say that you perform 1,000 arm movements or other reaching activities that are in the red zone. Including the weight of your arm, you are probably moving about 15,000 to 25,000 pounds in the red zone every day. These activities probably equate to 100,000 foot-pounds of torque more than would have been necessary if you had stayed in the green and yellow zones. No wonder you hurt worse as a typical day progresses.

If you could nearly eliminate red zone movements and minimize yellow zone movements as much as is feasible, you would be able to sharply reduce your musculoskeletal strain and foot-pounds of torque moved throughout the day, perhaps by more than 50 percent, and accomplish the same amount. How much less pain would you have? If you further minimized bending, stooping, and twisting, how much less pain would you have? When my patients commit to this strategy, they find that their average pain decreases about twenty points on a scale of 0-100!

HOW BAD WALKING MECHANICS CAN INCREASE PAIN

Physical activity includes not only specific movements like lifting, carrying, bending, or stooping, but also the more general postures of standing, walking, sitting, and lying down. How you perform these gross body movements can affect your pain tremendously throughout the day. For many people in pain, improper standing and walking mechanics may be the single major contributor to pain.

Standing for an extended length of time increases almost any type of skeletal or neuromuscular pain. It can be helpful to shift your weight from side to side. In your kitchen, you may be able to open a floor-level cabinet and place one foot on the ledge a little off the ground. You may want to keep a footstool handy that you can alternate resting your legs on. The stool will also help you lift objects that are high enough to be in the red zone. Frequent breaks from standing may be important even if you just walk around for a few seconds.

Your Walking Posture

Most of my patients have terrible walking mechanics that contribute to their pain. Let's begin with the classic walking posture taught to young women years ago and marines now. Head is up, chest out, stomach in, shoulders back, and able to balance a book on your head. It turns out that this is terrible posture and contributes strongly to spine and knee pain.

With your head up all the way, you increase the flexion in your neck, which tightens muscles, and places more strain on your cervical discs. With chest out and shoulders all the way back, you increase the flexion or lordosis (curvature) in your lumbar spine, which increases low back pain. These mechanics also tend to produce a straight-legged walking style. This allows you to balance a book on your head because you are not bending your legs or moving up and down much, but it makes your spine and joints support your weight rather than your muscles. That unhealthy walking style produces much greater stresses and impact on your bones, spinal discs, and connective tissue with each step you take.

Think about walking from an evolutionary perspective with humans as "great apes." Apes are referred to as "knuckle draggers" in part because they walk with strongly bent knees while moving their shoulders back and forth with their palms facing backward and their knuckles forward. In contrast, when you hold your shoulders rigidly back with chest out, your palms naturally face sideways, toward each other.

Healthier walking occurs when your shoulders are slightly rounded, just enough that your palms are facing backward, like the knuckle-dragging apes. The upper torso should not be rigid but should move fluidly with the walking motion. Your head should be naturally canted down slightly, such that your eyes are pointing toward the ground about ten yards in front of you, neither at the sky, nor at your feet.

Of equal importance as you walk, your knees should remain bent a little as you step, so that much of your weight is supported by your quadriceps, the muscle at the top of your thigh. This decreases spinal lordosis or curvature and provides some cushioning for the pounding of each step taken. Your head will naturally go up and down somewhat as your knees bend and straighten.

Finally, your weight should shift slightly from side to side with the majority of your weight, or center of gravity over the foot that is on the ground, not over the midline of your body. Many people walk the way that two-year-olds ice skate—with straight legs, little steps, and a wide, shuffling gait that keeps the center of gravity over the midline of the body. Notice how a world-class ice skater like Michelle Kwan moves. Most of the time, she is on one skate with all her weight on that one skate. The mechanics of walking also work best when the weight shifts almost completely from one foot to the other. Putting all the above walking mechanics together, you would not easily be able to balance a book on your head.

Pronating

Your feet are a critical part of your walking mechanics. With a normal, healthy step, your heel hits the ground first, followed by the outside or knife-edge of the foot connected to the little toe. As the knee moves forward over the foot, the foot literally rotates from the outside edge to the inside edge so the entire foot from heel to the ball of the foot can contact the ground. This rotation is called pronating and is at the core of the proper mechanics of walking. As the knee moves forward of the toes, the weight has shifted from the outside edge to the inside edge, and you push off the ground with the big toe.

Some people usually do not pronate enough because they have long, skinny, rigid feet with high arches. This under-pronating is also called supinating and can cause various problems with the feet and ankles as well as knees, hips, and spine. Supinators will show a wear pattern on the bottom of their shoes with almost all the wear on the outside edges of both feet, especially the heels.

Some people pronate too much, which is referred to as over-pronating. They tend to have very flexible feet that are often short and squat with low arches. This type of foot mechanic can also cause problems with knees, hips, and spine. The wear pattern of over-pronators will show heavy wear on the inside edge of both shoes, especially near the ball of the foot. People who pronate "just right" are called neutral pronators or biomechanically blessed or Goldilocks, take your pick. They are less likely to develop additional orthopedic problems.

The Importance of Selecting Shoes for Specific Walking Styles

It is important for you to know your pronating pattern. Each unique brand and style of shoe is made primarily for only one of the three walking styles. Formal walking or running shoes are constructed very specifically for only one of the three patterns. Shoes for supinators are usually heavily cushioned and highly flexible to encourage ankle and foot rotation. Shoes for over-pronators tend to be less cushioned and more rigid. They may even have a piece of plastic or metal along the inside edge of the shoe to minimize pronation. Neutral pronators wear shoes that are moderately cushioned and a little more rigid, but without the inner edge stabilization.

Good walking or running shoes can be found in many specialty stores and some regular clothing stores. Experienced staff should know whether a shoe is made for a pronator or supinator or for a heavy or light person. Heavier people need more cushioning regardless of pronation style. With running shoes, the rule of thumb is to replace them every 500 miles.

Walking shoes that you wear several times per week should probably be replaced about once a year. Don't be shy about spending extra money on shoes. Good shoes and good mattresses are the two most important purchases you will make if you have chronic pain. Rockport makes an excellent, modestly priced shoe that had the original patent on the Vibram sole, which set the standard for outstanding cushioning. Mephisto also makes an excellent shoe, although more expensive than Rockport, they carry a lifetime warranty.

If you do a lot of walking or running, notice the types of surfaces you use. Generally, the softer the surface, the better it is for your body. Hard-packed sand and level grassy areas are excellent. Dirt trails or roads are next best. Black asphalt roads are better than concrete sidewalks. Try not to do all of your walking on concrete. Mix up your surfaces a little. Most treadmills are quite soft. Marble floors are not very forgiving. You may notice that walking up and down hills is more painful than walking on level surfaces.

How Improved Sitting Posture Can Decrease Pain

Many people in pain spend much more time sitting during the day than standing or walking. Generally, good sitting posture means ninety-degree angles everywhere. Your back should be straight up and down making a ninety-degree angle at your hips with your thighs, which should be parallel to the ground. Your thighs should make a ninety-degree angle at the knees with your legs. Your legs should make a ninety-degree angle at the ankles with your feet, which are flat on the floor. Your heels should be directly below and in line with your knees. Your elbows should be directly below and in line with your shoulders. Your hands should be resting comfortably either in your lap or with one hand on each thigh. In a perfect world, your lower back is against the chair, a pillow or other support.

Many people in pain sit in a much-distorted manner. Depending upon which body parts hurt, you may push your buttocks forward in the chair so you look like you are almost lying down. You may sit partially sideways with one buttock on the chair and the other raised slightly. Or, you may place your hands on one or both arms of the chair to help support your weight. While these postures develop as a way of bracing and guarding against the pain, over the long run, they will increase your pain.

It is nearly impossible to sit healthily in a chair that does not fit you well. If the chair seat is too high or too low, your thighs and legs may not be able to make a ninety-degree angle and you may hurt worse. If the chair is too high, you can use a stool or books to rest your feet on. If the seat is too deep from back to front, it will tend to force your legs and feet outward and your low back away from the back of the chair. This can be corrected slightly by using a cushion or other support.

The back of the chair may be too short or too tall with the latter forcing your head forward. The average chair is made for someone about 5' 10" tall. If you are much taller or shorter, you may have trouble with most chairs. Examine the chairs and couches in your own home. Which ones fit you the best and which ones are worse? Are the couches so soft that you disappear into them and cannot maintain good posture? Are the chairs so hard they make you hurt after a short time? You may consider purchasing better-fitted chairs or couches. How about the seat in your car? With this new information, could you adjust your car seat so that it fits you better?

HOW TO DECREASE PAIN WHILE LYING DOWN OR SLEEPING

On average, people spend a third of their lives lying down with the vast majority of that time in bed. You will remember that if you have pain, your mattress and your shoes are the most important purchases you will make. If your mattress is more than ten years old, you need a new one. People in pain will argue whether a firm or soft mattress is best, with waterbeds being the ultimate in soft mattresses.

In television commercials, you may see a curving body on top of a mattress that also curves to support the body at all points; this was the original idea of the waterbed. However, if you have chronic pain that is skeletal or neuromuscular, then your body is likely distorted in some way that probably worsens over the course of the day. Do you want a mattress that conforms to your distorted body or a mattress that gently encourages your body to be less distorted, to conform to a healthier position? Naturally, you want a firmer mattress that encourages your body to be less distorted.

Most mattress manufacturers have a firmness gradient for the types of mattresses they sell and you should probably purchase one that is extra firm or firm. Often, very firm mattresses have a pillow top. This topper is a few inches thick and provides extra softness and cushion for the underlying firm mattress. There are excellent, new-generation mattresses, such as Tempur-pedic®, a spring-less mattress that provides firm support and comfort through dense foam that feels like heavy angel food cake. Developed with NASA astronauts in mind, these mattresses are expensive, but probably the best in the world for people in pain.

It is important to know in which position you sleep, whether on your side, back, or stomach. For most people with pain, it is healthiest to sleep on your back. If you have traditionally been a stomach sleeper, you should sleep on your side or back by trying to fall asleep on your back and restricting your turning movement with pillows, covers, etc.

Ultimately, the thickness of the pillow you select will be based upon your sleeping position. If you are a back sleeper, you will want your pillow to compress to about two inches thick. A side sleeper should have a pillow that compresses to about four inches thick. Fiercely independent and noncompliant stomach sleepers should minimize pillow thickness as much as possible. Fortunately, many pillow manufacturers label their pillows for side or back sleepers. Stomach sleepers are punished and don't get their own pillows.

Sometimes, the position in which you fall asleep is not the position in which you stay asleep. It can be helpful to ask a sleeping partner in which position you normally sleep. Depending on the specifics of your pain problem, you might also benefit from a body pillow or wedge that you can place between your knees. Some people have less pain if they place a wedge or pillows under their legs if they sleep on their back. This reduces the curvature of the spine and can decrease spine pain.

Improving your posture, body mechanics, and ergonomics will decrease your pain, and you will be able to accomplish activity that is more physical throughout the day. These changes are effortful and demand a scientific approach to your lifestyle. However, the rewards are inevitable if you choose to change.

Healthy body mechanics and ergonomics will decrease my pain

Insight—I can become more aware of my posture and body mechanics.
Commitment—I am committed to improving my posture while sitting, standing, and lying down and keeping my activities mostly in the green zone.
Action—I will evaluate the ergonomics of my home, bed, and shoes.
Now—I will freeze my posture in this moment, assess it, and make the necessary healthy changes.

14

Forty-Five Seconds to Relaxation

Relaxation is vital regardless of your health or life situation. Chronic stress and tension, hard work, and guilt over "being lazy" can impair your ability to relax, to wash away past mistakes, daily hassles, and future fears. Relaxation techniques can decrease your global nervous system arousal and anxieties to help you better manage stress. They can also decrease muscle tension, the most common trigger for increased chronic pain.

A key element of relaxation training is differentiating between being relaxed and being sleepy. Most of us equate the two. Not surprisingly, in times of stress and sleep deprivation, you may find that when you are relaxed you tend to fall asleep. This is natural and can be used as a sleep aid, but you also need to be able to relax in a wakeful, alert state. Chronic tension should not be your body's way of saying, "Okay, I'm awake now." Being able to relax is a skill you can learn. However, it will be necessary to practice relaxation on a regular basis, as you would any newly learned skill. This can help make it a healthy habit.

You should incorporate relaxation training into your rehabilitation program and relaxation techniques into your daily life. There are dozens of widely recognized relaxation strategies that might be helpful for you. Traditionally, learning relaxation techniques first involves learning how to completely relax by going through structured, lengthy exercises for fifteen to thirty minutes or longer. Once you are competent in knowing how to fully relax, you can learn techniques that take less time, as short as five to ten seconds. It may not be necessary to employ longer relaxation exercises on a daily basis for the rest of your life. Nevertheless, it is helpful to practice these longer techniques daily for a month and then taper to weekly for a year.

THE CLEANSING BREATH IS THE KEY TO ALL RELAXATION

Diaphragmatic breathing is the most common of all relaxation exercises and usually the most important. Healthy, effective breathing comes from the diaphragm. It makes the stomach go up and down with each breath as air is pushed almost completely in and out of the lungs on each breath. Exchanging air at the bottom of the lungs is referred to as deep breathing. Many of us get into the habit of shallow breathing, which means exchanging air only at the top portion of the lungs closest to the mouth. This breathing style makes the chest go up and down, not the stomach.

A simple way to allow yourself to breath diaphragmatically is to exhale gently, but forcefully, through your mouth until you have no more breath left. Then, inhale through your nose as deeply as you can. Most people prefer to start with the deep breathing in and then follow with the deep breath out. The "cleansing breath" is based upon this strategy. Breathe in slowly and deeply through your nose, counting 1, 2, and 3. When you cannot breathe in any more, exhale through your mouth while counting 1, 2, 3, 4, 5 slowly until you cannot comfortably exhale any more. Then gently and normally breathe in. Try a cleansing breath now—in through the nose 1, 2, 3, and out through the mouth 1, 2, 3, 4, 5. Now through the nose, breathe in and out, as you normally would.

Did you get a little head rush? Most people do. You are probably not accustomed to breathing in and out deeply and fully. However, the more you practice this, the less "buzzed" you will feel each time. The cleansing breath is a cornerstone for pain control within your Personal Pain Paradigm. You should take a cleansing breath several dozen times a day. Besides calming you and settling your thoughts, it is a signal that a change in thought, feeling, or behavior is to follow.

When you pace yourself and you switch activities or postures, you should take a cleansing breath. Any time you want to stop an unhealthy thought, you can take a cleansing breath. When you feel any intense negative emotion, you can begin changing the feeling with a cleansing breath. Whenever you feel afraid, you can repeat cleansing breaths frequently.

Many people in pain wrestle with intense anxiety, especially during periods of severe pain. This can include racing thoughts, rapid heart beat, palpitations, shortness of breath, or chest tightness, all symptoms of high anxiety or low-grade anxiety attacks. At these times, you may notice that it feels difficult to breathe, especially to inhale. You might be surprised to learn that the problem is really with your exhaling, and not with your inhaling.

In a moment, I want you to take a deep breath in through your mouth. You will hold the breath for a second without exhaling. Then take another deep mouth breath in without having exhaled from the first breath. Hold this breath a second and again, without exhaling, try to take a third deep breath in and hold it for a second. Then exhale completely and breathe normally. That's three breaths in with no breaths out until after the third breath. Got it? Okay.

Now, breathe in deeply and fully and hold 1. Breathe in again and hold 2. Then, try to breathe in a third time and hold 3. Now exhale fully and breathe normally. It's hard to take that second breath in, isn't it? And harder still to take the third one, because your lungs are already full of air. It does not really matter whether the air in your lungs is oxygen or carbon dioxide. The beach ball will not take more air without popping. Most times when you are short of breath, the key is to exhale fully and completely and then breathe in deeply. This feels almost crazily counterintuitive but it works well.

You can also try the cleansing breath exercise while you are exercising and your heart is really racing. Your breath is ragged in part because you need so much more oxygen in your lungs to support the various bodily demands. It is even more important to exhale completely, otherwise carbon dioxide builds up in your lungs, and you fatigue. This makes you have to stop and catch your breath. As a recreational runner for most of my life, I have used this strategy to calm my pounding heart. It really works.

HOW TO RELAX YOUR MUSCLES

Another strategy for relaxation is called progressive muscle relaxation. It is the gold standard and the grandfather of relaxation techniques. This involves tightening and relaxing individual body parts in a progressive sequence so you use all of the major muscle groups. You are trying to tighten the muscles beyond your chronic tension level and then fatigue them, so your post-progressive tension is less than at the beginning of the exercise.

Right now, sit in a comfortable, upright position with your feet flat on the floor, and try the following exercise. You will start at your toes, and successively tighten and relax body parts as you go up. Now begin and:

• Curl your toes and relax them

- Tighten your calves and relax

- Tighten your thighs and relax

- Tighten your buttocks and relax

- Tighten your stomach and relax

- Make a fist and relax

- Tighten your forearms and relax

- Tighten your biceps and relax

- Tighten your shoulders and relax

- Tighten your neck and relax

- Frown and relax your forehead

In many versions of this progressive relaxation, you clench and relax each body part three times before moving on to the next in the sequence. You can order progressive muscle relaxation compact discs through Amazon.com, or you can buy them at www.MyPainReliefDoc.com.

How the Body Scan Can Promote Relaxation

Another relaxation technique is called the body scan or autogenic training, which is often used in conjunction with other strategies, but can promote relaxation on its own. You can proceed from either the head down or the toes up.

For our purposes, we will perform this technique from the head down. Imagine your various body parts feeling heavy and relaxed. You can make slight movements if you want to—up and down, side to side, or twist and turn a little. The point is that you become mindful of your body parts in a sequential way, allowing any muscular tension to dissipate as best it can by simply letting go. In order from top down, become aware of being relaxed and heavy in:

- Your forehead

- Your jaw

- The back of your neck

- Your shoulders

- Your arms

- Your hands

- Your chest

- Your stomach

- Your back

- Your buttocks

- Your thighs

- The backs of your legs

- Your ankles

- Your feet

The body scan with autogenic training is a more passive relaxation technique than progressive muscle relaxation. It is less about doing and more about letting go, letting yourself relax, letting your thoughts quiet, letting your mind be in tune with your body.

FORTY-FIVE SECONDS TO RELAXATION THROUGH THE QUICK RELEASE

Over the years, I have developed a very effective progressive relaxation technique, called the Quick Release that incorporates the cleansing breath, a specific progressive muscle relaxation (PMR), and a body scan.

I have taught this technique to thousands of patients over the years and designed it for sitting or lying positions. The specific progressive muscle relaxation begins with your feet flat on the ground, and sitting up in the correct posture position of ninety-degree angles that you learned in Chapter 12. Try the sequence of tension and movements listed below as you read them. You should complete each action and after each one, you will relax back to neutral posture.

- Curl your toes

- Uncurl them

- Lift the balls of your feet and your toes toward the ceiling with your heels on the ground. (You will feel tension in your calves)

- Now drop the balls of your feet back down

- Push down on your heels (You will feel tension in your upper thighs)

- Now relax your heels

- Tighten your buttocks

- Now relax your buttocks

- Tighten your stomach by pushing down and out

- Relax the stomach

- Push down toward the ground with your elbows (tension in shoulders, upper arms)

- Relax and return elbows to normal position

- Pull your hands back and push your palms forward (tension in lower arms and hands)

- Relax and return hands to normal position

- Push your chin straight forward (tension in back of your neck)

- Return chin to baseline position

- Tilt your head up (tension in throat and clavicle area)

- Tilt head back down

- Grit your teeth (tension in jaws and lower face)

- Ungrit your teeth and relax your jaw

- Frown (tension in forehead)

- Stop frowning

With each of these movements in the PMR, you will feel tension in one or more body areas. See if you can tighten these areas further through isometrics, pitting one muscle group against another. If you are not sure how to do that, you can learn by trying the next exercise.

ISOMETRIC EXERCISE

Press your palms together in front of you with palms facing and fingers straight up or straight out. Each finger of one hand is pressed against the corresponding finger on the other hand. Now press your hands together as hard as you can without hurting yourself. See if you can maintain that tension while slowly pulling your hands an inch or two apart from each other so they no longer touch. You do this by way of isometrics, invisibly pitting one muscle group against another in the same body part.

As you tighten each body part in the PMR, you can add an isometric exercise to that body part to tighten it even more. Run through this palm-pressing exercise a few times before we proceed to the next technique.

QUICK RELEASE RELAXATION TECHNIQUE

The Quick Release technique combines the PMR, a cleansing breath, and a body scan into a powerful forty-five second relaxation exercise that can decrease anxiety, tension, moodiness, obsessive thoughts, or pain. First, I will describe what you do and then we will proceed through an actual exercise.

You take a cleansing breath to settle yourself and then you perform the progressive muscle relaxation, except this time you do not relax after tightening each body part. You maintain the tension in each successive body part until your entire body is tense, hold the tension for three seconds, then release the tension for three seconds. You take another cleansing breath and as you breathe in, raise your shoulders upward toward your ears while feeling your whole body seem to lift up, off the chair. Then as you exhale, you drop, drop, drop your shoulders. After dropping your shoulders, you begin a body scan, beginning with your forehead and ending with your feet, releasing even more any leftover tension in your body.

At the end of the body scan, you take one more cleansing breath. Breathing is normal at all times unless you are taking a cleansing breath. The second and third cleansing breaths are less vigorous than the one before it. As you learn this exercise, only tense up your body about 30 percent as tight as you can. Let's try the Quick Release now.

Take a cleansing breath by breathing slowly and deeply through your nose counting 1, 2, 3. Then, exhale through your mouth while counting 1, 2, 3, 4, 5 slowly until you cannot comfortably exhale anymore. Then gently and normally breathe in. Take several more breaths that are normal. Now comes the progressive muscle relaxation part of this exercise.

1. Curl your toes

2. Lift the balls of your feet and your toes toward the ceiling with your heels on the ground

3. Push down on your heels

4. Tighten your buttocks

5. Tighten your stomach by pushing down and out

6. Push down toward the ground with your elbows

7. Pull your hands back and push your palms forward

8. Push your chin straight forward

9. Tilt your head up

10. Grit your teeth

11. Frown

12. Hold the tension for three seconds, 1, 2, 3.

13. Then release, release, let go 2, 3, 4.

14. Take another cleansing breath, and as you breathe in, lift your shoulders up, up, up and then exhale, and drop, drop, drop, your shoulders.

15. Now begin a body scan. Move, jiggle, and turn as you want. Feeling heavy and warm is:

- Your forehead
- Your jaw
- The back of your neck
- Your shoulders
- Your arms
- Your hands
- Your chest
- Your stomach
- Your back
- Your buttocks
- Your thighs
- The backs of your legs
- Your ankles
- Your feet

16. Now, take one more cleansing breath—slower, softer, calmer, and breathe normally.

When you are not trying to complete this exercise by reading it in a book, it works better with your eyes closed, especially when it comes to the body scan. If you are doing this in public, you may want to skip the neck forward and chin up parts. They make you look weird. At least that's what people tell me when I do it.

The Quick Release takes about forty-five seconds and incorporates techniques from five relaxation exercises into a synergistic process of surrendering tension and stress. If you practice this a dozen times a day for a week or two, you will become an expert at it and it will become second nature to you.

In the past twenty years, I have performed the Quick Release over 10,000 times. I find that when I get to the body scan, I tend to have leftover tension in my shoulders, stomach, and back of my legs that I then have to release further. The Quick Release has become like an old friend, a quiet time for me, a reward for hard effort and perseverance.

RELAXATION HELP THROUGH BIOFEEDBACK TRAINING

Some people find it difficult to learn relaxation from a book, tape, or compact disc. You may need additional professional help. Biofeedback therapists specialize in relaxation training using their computer-based equipment and their own education and training. Traditionally, biofeedback for relaxation training has used sensors that measure skin temperature, sweating response, and muscle tension. All of these are indices of anxiety and corresponding autonomic nervous system arousal. Skin temperature is usually measured on the index fingertips of both hands. When you are anxious, the blood vessels in your skin, especially hands and feet, constrict such that the surface temperature of the skin gets colder. This can also reflect poor circulation as in Raynaud's Syndrome or peripheral neuropathy from diabetes.

The more anxious you are, the more your skin perspires, especially the palms of your hands, which make them conduct electricity better. Electrodermal activity is usually measured on the palms of the hands with higher readings associated with greater anxiety.

Increased muscle tension is associated with increased arousal and anxiety. Most people demonstrate the greatest muscle tension changes from stress in the forehead (frontalis muscle) and the neck where it leads into the shoulder (trapezius muscle). EMG levels are usually taken at these sites with higher levels reflective of greater tension and corresponding stress.

Usually a biofeedback therapist will establish baseline arousal levels for you in a normal state, a relaxed state, and a cognitively stressed state. Initially, the goal is to help you recognize how differences in anxiety and stress levels feel. Then, the therapist will explore multiple relaxation techniques that may include diaphragmatic breathing, progressive muscle relaxation, autogenic training, self-hypnosis, or guided imagery.

Biofeedback training is one of the most important components of a comprehensive pain program. Inevitably, the biofeedback therapist can help you reliably produce physiological changes in posture, gait, body mechanics, and general relaxation that decrease your pain. I have also heard every excuse not to meet with the biofeedback therapist, most of which were lies covering up the adage: "I will lie down here and let you do anything to me, but don't ask me to learn to help myself."

Biofeedback is not mind over matter. It is not something that is only helpful if you are weak-willed or not in "real" pain. It is not related to your pain tolerance. The fact that you are a tough police officer or were a Marine in "The War" is irrelevant. It is not the devil's handiwork, and does not violate the scriptures of any known religion. In the kind and gentle words of my former mentor, "Get on with it."

Relaxation exercises should be an element of my self-management

Insight—I understand the importance of performing regular relaxation exercises.
Commitment—I am committed to learning and practicing relaxation techniques including the Quick Release.
Action—I will do the Cleansing Breath repeatedly throughout the day to signal changes in thoughts, feelings, and behaviors.
Now—I will do a Cleansing Breath right now and at the end of each chapter.

15

Choosing Your Daily Activity Pattern with Chronic Pain

We have discussed that reasonable goals for people in pain are to decrease pain, increase activity, or both. Further, we have divided into five categories the types of activities that people spend their time on during an average sixteen-hour waking day:

- Physical

- Pleasurable

- Social

- Productive

- Rest

For people in pain, we would like to minimize your pain and maximize the amount of healthy time spent in non-resting activity. Let's continue developing your Personal Pain Paradigm, and look at your activity pattern before and after your pain problem developed.

CHARTING YOUR PHYSICAL ACTIVITY PATTERN IN A TYPICAL DAY

Physical activities include walking, standing, or even sitting if you are using your arms. Pleasurable activities are fun or enjoyable. You would do them for free.

Social activities are those that involve interacting with other people. Productive activities are those activities necessary for living or giving you a sense of accomplishment, such as paid work, cleaning the house, or running errands. Rest can be anything from lying down, to vegging on the couch in front of the TV, to reading a book.

Many activities overlap several categories. For example, going for a walk with a friend might be physical, social, and pleasurable. Cleaning out the garage might be both physical and productive. Take a moment right now, and in your TAAP journal, write down the percentage of time you typically spent in each of the five categories in a sixteen-hour waking day before you had pain. Then total your score for the four activities other than rest. Your total score will probably add up to more than 100 because so many activities overlap several categories. List the hierarchical order of activities from most time to least time spent in a typical day before you had pain.

Now do the same task for the period since you have experienced pain, especially your activity levels in the past three months. Write down the percentage of time you have spent in each of the five categories in a typical day and total the four non-rest activities again. Now, list the hierarchical order of activities from most time spent to least time spent in a typical day after you had pain.

Compare your pre-and post-pain activity lists. Which activities changed the most? Which changed the least? How is the order of activities different? How much did your total activity levels change? Are there any surprises for you here?

I have been using this activity assessment for many years with my patients, and some definite trends have emerged. Not surprisingly, the total activity level (not counting rest) drops dramatically after chronic pain develops, usually by about two-thirds or more. Before pain developed, physical and productive activities were usually the highest scores, followed by social and then pleasurable activity. Rest is minimal before pain onset and virtually always the lowest score.

After the onset of pain, rest usually goes from lowest score to about the highest score for those patients not still gainfully employed. The remaining activities after the onset of pain are usually ordered as productive, physical, social, and pleasurable. Note that the order of non-rest activities is often similar before and after pain, but people engage in much less of each of the non-rest activities after pain onset.

Additionally, the specific productive and physical activities being performed have changed dramatically. You may have gone from working as a floor nurse twelve hours per day to tidying up the house six hours per day. Even within the six hours you are physically active, your activity is much less physically demanding and rewarding. Most people report that the non-rest activities with the highest percentage change are social and pleasurable.

Before pain onset, people usually have the attitude that time was the only thing that limited what they could do. Physically healthy people usually have a lot of energy. They can be tired but get second and third winds when needed. During particularly busy periods, they can even steal time from sleeping to create more than sixteen waking hours in a day. Many people pride themselves on being able to be on the go constantly, in motion all the time, able to combat sleep deprivation and still function.

All those things change after pain starts. There may be plenty of time in a day, but too much pain and not enough energy. You know that there is only so much non-rest activity that you can accomplish in a day, before you begin to crash from pain and fatigue. There are severe limits to second and third winds. Sleep deprivation inevitably makes your pain worse with a fatigue that may be too great to overcome, regardless of your motivation.

When you have pain, you need to organize your activities in the healthiest way, one that maximizes your quality of life and your ability to get things done. When you hurt, you must restructure your activities and focus a little less on units of time and a little more on units of energy. You may have six hours after your child or spouse comes home, but no energy left for big projects. In this situation, time is irrelevant.

Certainly, good pacing and limit setting will help you maximize your activities, but you need to plan for it. If you have 100 energy units to spend during the day, how will you budget them? As you set goals and begin to arrange the structure for your day, how will you apportion your energy between rest and non-rest, e.g., physical, social, pleasurable, and productive activities? What will most improve your quality of life? What will help you feel like you are accomplishing things? What will help you manage your pain the best?

How Distracting Activities Can Decrease Pain

Into this discussion of healthy activities, we add the concept of activities that distract from pain. I have asked every pain patient I have ever evaluated how he or she copes with pain. The two most common responses are "pain pills" and "I just keep going." Both of these are unhealthy responses for different reasons. The more you use pain pills to manage pain fluctuations, the less you are using and learning long-term self-management strategies. "I just keep going" usually means you try not to think about it much and try to live your life the same way you always have. However, even moderate pain will not let you live your life the way you always have.

You need to structure your life with pain in a way that scientifically and deliberately distracts you from hurting. Distraction techniques and distracting activities are often categorized as either active or passive. Initially, you might think of active as physically active and so believe that active distraction would include things like walking, bicycling, or doing chores. Passive distraction is viewed as things like reading a book, watching television, or listening to music.

However, the continuum of passive to active distraction actually means the extent to which an activity forcefully pulls your attention away from pain and toward the activity. Actively distracting events demand your mental participation so intensely that they fill your attention and leave room for little else. Walking across a balance beam suspended a few inches above a vat of acid to save your child on the other side would be actively distracting. Watching the grass grow in a meadow might be passive. Going for a walk is not necessarily distracting, since it leaves you free to obsess about how much you hurt, along with other darkly negative thoughts.

Talking to other people is an active distraction because they expect your full participation. You need to respond, ask questions, use eye contact, etc., all of which pulls your attention away from your pain. Walking with a friend is a great active distraction since your body and your mind are fully occupied. Playing video games can be an active distraction because you must focus intensely to proceed through the game.

Talking on the phone is a less active distraction than talking in person since you are not responsible for your body language. Many of us pride ourselves on being able to pay bills or care for our kids while we are talking to Aunt Ethel on the phone. You cannot do that in person. While an extremely good movie may grab your attention and not let go for a while, the myriad of mindless shows on television may not grab you as much. Who hasn't been so engrossed in their own thoughts while watching television that they could not explain the plot when someone came into the room and asked, "What's this show about?" Reading is another relatively passive distraction since most of us have experienced times that we could not remember what we had just read in the previous few pages.

You have already assessed how much of your recent time has been spent in the various activities and during rest periods. Review a typical day again with an eye toward how effectively you distract yourself from pain. If most of your time is spent indoors, alone, and reading, watching television, or playing on the computer, then you are probably spending way too much time thinking about your pain and associated misery. You need to start planning for more distractions that are active.

How to Improve Your Ability to Distract Yourself from Pain

Using distraction effectively to help manage pain requires good attention and concentration. Even with the more active distractions that draw your attention, you need to be able to concentrate for a certain period of time. The longer you have hurt and the more time you spend in passive distraction, the weaker your concentration skills become. However, you can strengthen them using the STAR and STIM techniques. With Sensory Training at Rest (STAR), you can practice concentration by observing an object intensely for 30-180 seconds and making as many observations about it as you can. Try not to relate the object to yourself with judgments like good, pretty, talented, comforting, etc. Try to focus purely on what you see, hear, or smell. Set up a dialogue with yourself, a running commentary that you sub-vocalize that is more than just rapid thinking. Use a timer. You may find that you fatigue quickly. Your attention span is the length of time it takes you to have the first non-observational thought after beginning the exercise.

Sensory Training in Motion (STIM) is a more integrating way to practice concentration and actually a better distraction in itself. Here, you can move about your environment and again set up a running commentary in your head. Try to incorporate all five of your senses—sight, sound, touch, smell, and taste. You can pick things up and touch things. You can do this almost anywhere—the mall, the woods, or a doctor's office, though outdoors is usually best. Your task is to really notice and get in touch with your environment, to interact with it, not just passively move through it. You want to get out of "your head" and your past miseries to experience your world now as intensely as possible.

You should practice the STAR and STIM techniques on a regular basis. You may want to begin them with a cleansing breath or with the Quick Release relaxation process. In addition to practicing concentration, using the STAR and STIM strategies can help you break a cycle of negative obsessing, fear, or anger. They allow you to stop thoughts that are unhealthy or that make you miserable. They are effective, active distractions for pain.

A scientific approach to activity and distraction can increase my activity

Insight—I understand the value of managing my activities wisely with limited energy.

Commitment—I am committed to increasing physical, social, pleasurable, and productive activity.

Action—I will practice the STAR and STIM techniques to improve my attention and concentration to use distraction better.

Now—Right now, I will complete a STAR exercise by focusing on something in this room, and that thing is: _____.

16

How to Manage and Enjoy Social Activity

Of the four types of non-resting activities, socializing is the best distraction from pain. Why, then, do you tend to decrease your socializing time more than any other activity? Most likely, it is because it is so distracting. It takes tremendous energy to engage in an activity that demands your attention and participation. When you socialize, you interact, respond, and are responsible for what you say and do. The demands of leaving your home, driving somewhere, and being moderately entertaining for hours can feel overwhelming if you mainly want to curl up in bed. When people hurt over a long time, they tend to avoid and withdraw from everyone, even the people living with them.

HOW TO SOCIALIZE MORE WITH LESS FOCUS ON PAIN

Socializing is not just healthy because it is a distraction. One of the most common complaints I hear from patients who have pain for years is that they have lost most or all of their friends. Loneliness is almost synonymous with pain. People in pain complain that their friends do not want to be around them now that they are hurting and cannot come out and play the way they used to play. Sometimes this is true, but the real problem may be that the person in pain has declined offers to socialize so many times that the friends have stopped calling.

Many people in pain will acknowledge that they do not plan activities in advance, because they cannot know how they are going to feel on a given day, and do not want to renege at the last minute. This reasoning has caused the death of countless friendships and the destruction of millions of social support systems. To socialize more comfortably, you need to build a social network that can

166

accommodate your pain condition. You can probably do this with your existing family and friends, but you will need to mold them.

Another common complaint I hear is that people in pain hate socializing because they get tired of being asked about their pain problem, and even more tired of trite or pat suggestions about what to do to improve their situation. I have worked with several thousand family members of people with pain. In most cases, friends and non-spousal relatives ask questions about your pain partly because they are interested, partly because they feel obligated, and partly because they assume it will be better than the last time they asked. But, they really do not know what to say about your pain. It probably makes them feel awkward and uncomfortable, much like you might feel at a funeral talking to the spouse of the deceased. What do you say to make it better?

You cannot help your family and friends cope well with your pain condition until you become committed to coping better with your pain condition. Most importantly, you must accept your pain problem as chronic and long-term. You must not refer to yourself or think about yourself as being "sick." You are not sick. You have pain. So do sixty to eighty million other Americans and probably a billion people worldwide. You should minimize pain behaviors. You need to have topics of conversation other than pain and its consequences.

HOW TO MAKE YOUR SOCIAL SYSTEM MORE COMFORTABLE WITH YOUR PAIN

You can help your closest friends and family to structure their interactions with you in a healthy way. You can talk to them one at a time. You can say that the doctors have told you that they can't cure, or get rid of your pain problem, and you will probably have some pain and limitations for the rest of your life. If it seems appropriate, you can mention the multifactoral aspect of pain. You can say that your task is to manage the best you can with your condition, which means adjusting your life in a healthy way around your pain. This includes trying not to talk about it with other people. This will help you decrease your pain.

You can ask your support people to stop asking or talking about your condition so you can discuss it less. Tell them that the best support they can give you is to distract you as much as possible from your pain and understand if there are times when you are quiet, withdrawn, or a little snippy. Over time, you may have to remind them of these issues. If they persist, you might want to practice an assertion technique called "broken record" where you repeat a standard statement each time someone inquires about your pain. You can try a statement like, "I'm not supposed to talk about my pain," or "My doctors told me talking about my pain makes it worse."

It is important to be consistent and not send mixed messages to people. If there are young children in your life, age appropriate conversations are vital. They need to know that you are not sick, that you are not dying or going to die from your condition. They need to know that you will not be able to participate in certain activities, but that you can do other activities with them. They should be told that there might be times when you appear sad or angry, but you are not. They may need to know that none of this is their fault.

With family or friends that you see infrequently, you can skip long, drawn-out discussions and go to the broken record almost immediately by saying something like, "My doctors say I'm going to have to learn to live with it, and the more I talk about it the more miserable I'll be. So, I'm not supposed to talk about my pain."

How to Structure Socializing More Effectively

The expectations and demands of social interaction can make it the most difficult of all activities when you hurt. One of the goals of being forthright with your support system is to lower peoples' expectations of you. Maybe you do not want to be "up" and wildly gregarious when socializing. Maybe you will want to leave early or arrive late. Maybe you cannot participate in some of the activities. Perhaps you will need to take refresher breaks in which you go off by yourself for a little while. Maybe you need to sit down while talking. Each of these behaviors may represent a very different social you.

The Importance of Selfishness in Managing Social Interaction

My message to you is to ask for what you want. How could you structure a social event in a way that would make it most likely that you could participate? How can you be creative and flexible in organizing your interactions with others? By being up front about your condition, you normalize your pain for others and lower their expectations. This establishes the groundwork for making changes in how you interact with them and asking others for what you want.

Ask For What You Want

At first, it might be difficult to ask for what you want. Perhaps you think that it's inappropriate to ask because it breaks societal convention, it's inconvenient, or puts the other person in an awkward position. You might assume that you will not get what you want anyway, so why ask. You may have developed such a habit over many years of putting other people first that it simply does not occur to you to ask for what you want. You may have put other people first for so long that you do not even realize what you want much of the time. Effective self-management of chronic pain means taking care of yourself first.

Asking for what you want and molding the people around you are good examples of self-management as opposed to medical management of chronic pain. These strategies also reflect a necessary element in your Personal Pain Paradigm—selfishness. There is a supremely selfish aspect to managing pain that is necessary and inescapable.

Give Yourself Permission to Be Selfish

In every step toward managing pain better, you need to give yourself permission to be selfish. But, our society frowns on selfishness in spite of Ayn Rand's efforts to the contrary. Many of us define ourselves based upon how much we contribute to our loved ones, our community, or our church. We pride ourselves on giving more than we get. Being assertive or championing our own needs may feel very wrong, antithetical to our core identity as a giver. But, it is evident that with pacing, limit setting, goal setting, and structuring your environment, you will be putting yourself first. How do we resolve this conflict?

Perhaps you can reframe the issue by differentiating between the process and the outcome of self-management. A healthy paradigm of self-management means selfishly organizing your life in a manner consistent with some pain. You try to avoid situations that will compel you to manage your pain badly. However, the outcome of self-management includes both reduced pain and increased function, much of which you can direct toward other people. By selfishly minimizing your pain, you will leave yourself more energy and ability to give to others. If you continually push yourself beyond your limits, you will break down or deplete your reserves.

HOW YOU CAN BE A DESIRABLE SOCIAL PARTNER EVEN WITH PAIN

When your pain problem first developed, it was probably new and interesting. You may have felt a release in venting a little about your condition and treatments, and your support people may have rallied around you. Well, as the months and years have passed, it is no longer interesting and while you may seek their support, it's not helpful for them to rally around. You need to transition away from being "the guy with the bad back," or "the woman with Fibromyalgia." You do not want to be a walking, talking patient or advertisement for the failure of modern medicine everywhere you go. You do not want people to feel uncomfortable about what to say to you or how to treat you.

The more your life is consumed with pain, frustration, and medical appointments, the less likely you are to be an asset at a social gathering. To remain an interesting social person and allow your support system to help you, you need to have other things to discuss besides your pain. It's hard to act as if you have a life outside of medical appointments if you don't. You need to have or get a life outside of medical appointments and focus on that other life when you interact with family and friends. Watch the news, read the newspaper, take a class, volunteer somewhere, mentor someone, start writing your autobiography, develop a hobby, or continue to work. Pull things into your life that you can discuss besides your pain. We'll talk more about this later.

Practice Social Listening Skills

Talking with someone about something of interest to you is a great way to maintain friendships and distract yourself from pain. It combats the real and existential loneliness that people with pain often feel. It also requires a lot of energy. Listening, on the other hand, requires less energy, but it is not quite as good a distraction. While you are talking, you must work hard to say something modestly intelligent and related to the conversation.

When you are listening, you can space out or think about your pain or the broccoli stuck between their teeth. It is more work to talk than it is to listen. Since people love to talk about themselves, being a good socializer requires trying to be a better listener. Being a better listener makes listening a better distraction and makes socializing less effortful.

Social interaction is a free exchange of verbal and nonverbal communication between individuals and groups. Socializing involves making statements, giving information, and telling interesting stories. You can spend more time listening and become a better listener if you focus more on listening than talking. When you meet someone or talk to someone, adopt the attitude that your task is to learn something about or from this person that you didn't already know. Ask questions, especially open-ended questions that get the other person talking. Instead of saying, "Ya like the shrimp dip?" you could ask, "So, whattaya think's in the shrimp dip?" Instead of asking, "How do ya like school?" you could ask, "So, what classes are you taking in school?" If you know something the other person is interested in, ask open-ended questions about that.

Pain research has consistently demonstrated that one of the most important aspects of healthy pain management is social support. People with solid social support usually cope better with pain. If you already have an excellent support system, you have an advantage in learning self-management. If you do not have good support, creating a better support system is extremely important. There are people out there with similar interests or problems that would like to get to know you. You may need to take a risk and reach out. The rewards are worth it.

You can improve your socializing and ask for what you want

Insight—I understand that good self-management requires effective socializing.
Commitment—I am committed to improving my social skills as a person in pain.
Action—I will structure social situations in a healthier way by asking for what I want.
Now—One thing that would improve my social interactions is:

_____

_____

_____

_____

17

How to Communicate and Negotiate Better with Your Doctors

Social interaction is compromised when you have pain. You are probably distracted, miserable, and antsy, more focused on getting through it than getting something out of it. Your thoughts and words do not flow as well as they did before. It's harder to pay attention to what people are saying and to understand what they mean. Into this morass, we bring the issue of communication between you and your doctor. Poor patient-doctor communication is probably the greatest barrier to effective medical treatment.

Doctors almost inevitably think they communicate better than they do. They make a living talking to twenty to fifty patients a day. Many doctors give group lectures or symposiums. Patients, nurses, physical therapists, secretarial staff, drug reps, and others listen to the sage advice from the person at the top of the mountain, the doctor. Doctors are almost never questioned or confronted, and especially not about their communication, i.e., what they have said or how they said it. Primary care physicians in family practice, internal medicine, and gynecology tend to have the best communication skills. But, it is widely recognized that the more specialized physicians tend to communicate less well.

Doctors receive almost no training in communicating with patients. It is learned mostly on-the-job in residency and fellowship. The Western model of patient-physician interaction places primary responsibility on the doctor to understand and diagnose the problem and prescribe appropriate treatment. Doctor communication is designed mainly to glean information from the patient, not to give information to the patient. Providing patient information is almost a bonus, a throw away. Lengthy explanations interfere with the ability to move on to the next patient. The patient is expected to comply, but a patient's thorough understanding of the nature of his diagnosis is not particularly important in

Western medicine. The patient-physician interaction is complicated further by the brevity of the visits, on average ten to fifteen minutes per patient.

However, most pain patients do an even worse job of communicating than their doctors, especially compared to their communication skills in any other setting. I see bright, articulate, assertive, successful people turn into forgetful, mumbling, passive robots. Some doctors are models of patience and thoroughness. Others may come in appearing rushed and out of sorts. They may talk quickly, ask a few questions, mention a test or two, ask about prescription refills, and then leave, with the patient uncertain if the appointment is over or not.

GUIDELINES FOR TALKING TO DOCTORS DURING APPOINTMENTS

As a pain psychologist, I have talked to patients and their physicians thousands of time before, after, and sometimes during their appointments with each other. I would say that poor communication and misunderstanding by the patient is the rule, not the exception, and it is not necessary if patients will follow some simple guidelines.

Dr. Feelbetter is meeting with his patient, Iminpain, and the patient's spouse. He says, "I'm prescribing you Neurontin. That's 900 milligrams. We'll give you 300-milligram tablets three times a day, okay? I'll write the script and be right back."

Ten minutes later, a nurse hands the written prescription to the patient and then ushers the patient out. Neither the patient nor the spouse knows the dosing of the medicine, what benefits the patient may obtain, possible side effects, etc., but both hope the pharmacist will tell them.

The pharmacist asks the patient how long he's been having seizures. When the patient finds out that Neurontin is an anti-seizure medication, he walks out empty handed, refusing to pay for the medicine until he talks to the doctor again in six weeks. He is deeply disappointed and frustrated.

This is not only a true story but one lived by many patients. So, what daily dose and schedule do you think the doctor wanted the patient to take? Read the Dr. Feelbetter paragraph again. I'll wait.

Most people think the doctor prescribed Neurontin 300 mgs TID. That's one 300-milligram tablet of Neurontin taken three times per day for a total of 900 milligrams in a day. That conclusion would be wrong. The doctor actually prescribed Neurontin 300 mgs, 3 tabs, TID. That's three 300 milligram tablets of

Neurontin (900 mgs per dose) taken three times per day for a daily total of 2700 mgs of Neurontin. This is not a life-threatening misunderstanding but could have been with a different medication.

What the doctor said was technically accurate, but we can agree he communicated poorly. The real problem was that the patient did not confront the doctor and ask him to clarify the medication regimen. The situation was further complicated when the patient did not ask for additional information about the medication. Neurontin is in fact registered and marketed as an anti-convulsant, but is FDA approved for post herpetic neuralgia and heavily used "off label" for various neuropathic and sympathetically-mediated pain problems. It is a "cutting edge" medication for pain about which the pharmacist (or pharmacy technician) was uninformed.

Another patient was sent to me for psychological clearance for a spinal cord stimulator. This is the device we discussed in Chapter 1 that is implanted under the skin. It sends a vibrating electrical current down an arm or leg to mask or decrease nerve pain in the limb. The patient understood from talking to her physician that her pain would be eliminated and that her atrophied leg would become normal. Neither of these perceptions was accurate. The spinal cord stimulator would not eliminate her pain. At best, it would reduce it considerably. Since the technology of stimulation is not corrective, it would not directly affect her atrophy, except in making her better able to walk and probably helping her regain partial muscle strength. When informed of these facts, she tearfully declined to proceed with implantation.

How to Use Active Listening Techniques to Understand Your Doctors Better

In both cases above, the patients did not do an adequate job of information gathering and specifically did a poor job of listening. There is a well-established technique called "active listening" that can dramatically improve patient-physician communication. It is also called the four R's: repeat, rephrase, request, and respond.

First, you repeat what the doctor said word for word. "You're prescribing Neurontin. That's 900 milligrams. You'll give me 300-milligram tablets three times a day." The doctor says, "Right." Then you rephrase it in a way that makes sense to you. "So, I'll be taking 300 mgs three times a day for a total of 900 mgs daily." Then you request confirmation that your rephrasing was accurate by saying something like, "Did I get it right?" The doctor says, "No, that's not what I said. I want you to take 900 mgs three times a day for a total of 2700 mgs. Since the strongest tablet is only 300 mgs, you'll have to take three at a time."

If you are certain you understand, you can respond by asking a question like, "So, is 2700 mgs daily considered a lot?" Or, "What kind of medication is this?" Or, you could say, "I'll try the Neurontin for a month and see how it goes."

With an orthopedic surgeon, the conversation might go like this. "Well, I've reviewed your films and I think you need a lumbar fusion, but there's about an 80 percent chance of success and you're going back to work." You repeat, "An 80 percent chance of success and me going back to work." "Yep!" Rephrase the statement. "So, there's an 80 percent chance that I'll be pain free and able to do my old job?" Request a response. "Is that right?" The surgeon replies, "Well, not pain free, but at least you'll have less pain and function a lot better. But still, you probably could never return to your job as a professional wrestler."

Rephrase and Request again. "So there's an 80 percent chance I'll have less pain and be able to do more stuff, like working full-time at a less strenuous job. Is that right?" The surgeon answers, "Yep."

Now you could respond, "Is there a chance I could be worse off?" The physician might say, "Well, that's always a possibility." Now you have a much more realistic expectation of your surgical outcome. You can make a more informed decision and be more satisfied with your outcome when it results in less than complete recovery.

This active listening technique can and should be used in many social situations. This is a great way to make sure that you understand not just what the other person is saying, but what that person actually meant to say. This allows for other people in your life to communicate better and for you to discern what they really mean.

Using Your TAAP Journal during Appointments

Perhaps the most important element in communicating effectively with a doctor is to maintain a notebook that contains your discussions with the doctor and the questions that you intend to ask. Patients usually go to their pain doctors with questions, concerns, or new symptoms that they want to discuss. In many cases, they forget to bring up one or more of the issues because they were not written down.

It is also extremely helpful to write down what the doctor says in response to your questions or concerns. Practicing your active listening skills can help you ensure that what you are writing down is what the doctor meant. Writing down the answers to your questions also forces the doctor to slow down a little, which may be helpful if he is one of the speedy ones. At the beginning of your appointment, it is a good idea to tell the doctor, "I have five issues I'd like to discuss with you today." Your doctor will be frustrated if he thinks the appointment is over and then you come up with a list of issues.

You are responsible for your medical care and your treatment progress. You are also responsible for your medications, appointments, and communication with your doctor. You are not building trust or credibility when you come to an appointment with your spouse or support person who maintains all the pertinent information, meds, and appointment calendar, or who answers half or most of the doctor's questions. This permanently erodes your relationship with your doctor. You will inevitably have less credibility, be treated like a child or an elder, and find that your doctor ends up talking to the other person more than to you. You will lose your power and your autonomy. Quite frankly, you sacrifice respect. This is especially the case when the other person is a nurse case manager or has some legal standing like a conservator. You can avoid this by being the one who maintains all the information or by not having your support person attend all of your appointments.

Most physicians welcome questions—short, articulate, intelligent questions that are germane to your health and the reason for the visit. When they ask a question, they want a direct, brief, on-target answer. Then, you can add or embellish if you choose. One of the most frustrating things for a physician is working harder than he thinks he should have to. If your doctor asks you how many Vicodin you have left from your last prescription and you launch into a long story, it will not go over well. Answer his question, and then if you must, tell the story about the dog, the toilet, or the thieving gremlins.

MEDICAL TREATMENT IS A NEGOTIATION BETWEEN PARTNERS

Medical treatment planning is not merely a communication between patient and doctor. Rather, it is a negotiation. It should not always be a straightforward matter of the doctor dictating and you complying. That is fine if you consult your family practice doctor for a sinus infection. However, if you are actively involved in your pain care and you are developing your Personal Pain Paradigm, you will have preferences regarding your care and treatment selection. Part of the new covenant between you and your doctor that we discussed in Chapter 5 was to create a true partnership. Partners negotiate with each other.

For openers, ask for what you want. That should sound familiar. I have observed so many patients with a specific treatment request who never directly voice it. You waste time trying to maneuver the doctor into figuring out that she should recommend your desired treatment, and then you get frustrated when she does not recommend it. This happens most often when you fear that your request will make you look bad. Maybe you want stronger narcotics or more time off from work, but you do not want to accept responsibility for asking because you're concerned that you will appear to be drug seeking or lazy.

You can be direct about what you want and your doctor can disagree with you. Or, she can be direct about her recommendation and you can disagree with her. In either case, you might agree to follow her recommendation with the caveat that if it fails, you will proceed with your recommendation. Conversely, you might suggest that you want to proceed with your recommendation and if that fails, you will proceed with hers.

Keep in mind that it is often best to try only one new treatment at a time to ensure that changes in your condition can be attributed to a specific treatment. The length of time between appointments can be adjusted accordingly and is most certainly negotiable. But, make sure that your doctor knows what you want. She is responsible for how she receives this information. She can think whatever she wants.

You can ensure that your doctor understands what you want by asking her to practice active listening skills in a given situation. For instance, perhaps your doctor wants to terminate your physical therapy and you do not. She might say, "I think we should stop physical therapy." You might request that the doctor rephrase in her words your position on your physical therapy. You might say, "I'm not sure I did a good job of communicating how physical therapy has affected me. How do you understand what I said about it?" The doctor might reply with something like this, "Well, you said it wasn't helping you (rephrasing) so I think we should stop it." Then you can respond, "Actually, what I was trying to communicate was that my pain wasn't decreasing, but I am getting stronger with better endurance. I am able to do more things because of physical therapy and I'd like to continue for another month since pain relief isn't really the goal of physical therapy anyway." Here you are repeating and rephrasing what you originally said to the doctor and adding a compromise request. Naturally, the doctor appreciates her error and the wisdom of your negotiation and heartily agrees with you.

I will close this chapter with a few communication errors with doctors that you should avoid—garnered from several decades of my own clinical practice.

- Don't swear, yell, or threaten to sue and expect to stay in the doctor's practice.

- Don't use pain as an excuse for being rude.

- Don't stop the doctor in the hallway after your appointment for "just one quick question."

- Don't call the doctor the next day with a question you forgot to ask.

- Don't ramble when you talk.

- Don't accuse all your previous doctors of poor care. Your current doctor will figure she's next on your list.

- Don't be gracious and engaging with the doctor and a tyrant with her staff. She will find out.

- Don't demand special treatment; actually don't demand anything. Request and then justify.

I can improve my communication and negotiations with my doctors

Insight—I am responsible for understanding my doctor and communicating well with her.

Commitment—I am committed to communicating and negotiating more effectively with my doctor.

Action—I will practice the four R's of active listening with my doctors, family, and friends.

Now—One thing that I would like my doctor to try or do differently is:

_____
_____
_____
_____

18

How to Enhance Pleasurable Activity

Remember fun? It was that thing you used to do to reward yourself for working so hard. That would have been before the pain that seemed to suck the joy and happiness from your life. That was before having fun seemed like more effort than it was worth; before the pain that seems to make each day gray.

Pleasure is the dessert of life. It makes us feel good about ourselves and about living. Intensely pleasurable moments can feel like a justification for effort, for work, for struggle and suffering. Pleasure allows us to be kids again, to get back in touch with the childish part of ourselves. You can experience delight and simple joy from a walk through the woods, a ride at the fair, or eating an ice cream cone. Pleasure and fun beat back all the existential worries and shout at the Gods, "This is why I'm alive. This is why it's all worth it." Experiencing pleasure allows us to feel whole, integrated, and to be truly "in the now" with no thought of past failures or future worries. Experiencing pleasure is absolutely necessary for healthy function and life satisfaction.

Chronic pain drains pleasurable activities from life. This is the most insidious and quietly devastating of the losses caused by chronic pain. It seems obvious that pain will impact your physical activity. Your family and friends can attest that it affects social activity, but it is almost inevitable that chronic pain will change pleasurable activities, too. Maybe the best you can do is to minimize this negative change. Or, maybe you can still find joy even with pain.

The more physical were your pleasurable activities, the greater your loss from chronic pain. If you hiked regularly, played ball with your kids, rode bikes, spruced up your garden, or otherwise vigorously exercised, you may feel destroyed by your inability to do those things. On the other hand, if your idea of a good time was to lie on the couch and watch football all day, (nothing wrong with that) you can still probably do that even with pain. In fact, your pain condition may give you an excuse to do that, guilt free, on a regular basis.

WHAT ARE THE EFFECTS OF DECREASED PLEASURE FROM CHRONIC PAIN?

What happens when you do not engage in pleasurable activities anymore? What would happen if we took 100 people who were perfectly healthy and said to them, "For the next six months, you can do whatever you want, just nothing that is fun." A large percentage of those folks would end up clinically depressed.

Most people believe that depression is caused by really terrible events happening to them, usually one after the other. The truth is that lack of pleasurable activity, independent of terrible events, can cause depression. Not having fun contributes to existential anxiety, the "What's it all for?" question.

The Link between Depression and Chronic Pain

Depression and chronic pain are powerfully linked. Most people in pain attribute their depression to their pain. That may be true, but much of depression is caused by the sequelae of pain, including not being able to perform previously enjoyable activities. If you have chronic pain and are depressed, it is entirely possible that you would still be depressed if you did not have pain but were still avoiding previously pleasurable activity. It is vital that people with pain have fun. But how do you do that? You may need to modify the way you do enjoyable things.

Jim was a patient who was an excellent skier, having skied some of the most difficult hills on all the major slopes throughout the U.S. and Canada. Following a spine injury and surgery, he was advised to stop skiing due to the extreme demands on his spine and potential risks from falling. Unfortunately, this enjoyable activity formed the core of his social network and helped him manage stress. He decided that he could still ski the intermediate hills but would stay away from advanced (black diamond) hills. There would be much less twisting, turning, and impact from moguls, with less risk from falls. This would still allow him to have some fun and obtain all the other benefits he enjoyed so much.

STRATEGIES FOR INCREASING FUN WITH CHRONIC PAIN

Make a list of the activities you enjoyed in the year before your pain problem developed. Can you perform any of these activities in a modified way, perhaps less strenuously or with breaks? If you like to hike in the woods, you might stay on groomed trails, avoid steeply sloping hills, or rest frequently. If you like to bicycle, you might get a more cushioned mountain bike or adjust the seat and handlebars to promote a more upright posture with less reaching and bending. If you garden, you might spend some time thinking about how you can garden and stay more in the green and yellow reaching zones that we discussed earlier.

These are helpful suggestions that can genuinely improve the quality of your life, but lurking behind these helpful hints is some loss of passion. If you have a passion for your pleasurable activities, you may not want to modify or moderate them. The pure delight in these activities may be in the joyous, spontaneous abandon you feel when doing them. For instance, when you hike, you can go wherever you want, exploring as you choose, taking breaks when you want, and pushing yourself as much or as little as you want. Putting limits and boundaries on this activity may suck some of the joy out of it.

How to Be Moderate and Maintain Pleasure with Chronic Pain

I publish a free newsletter on my website at www.MyPainReliefDoc.com and had this to say about passion and moderation,

> "I hate being moderate. I hate doing things moderately. I hate having to be controlled, mature, and disciplined. I don't want to moderate how much I eat or drink. I don't want to be moderate with sex, playing, or vacations. I don't want to moderate what I say for fear it will offend. I don't want to do what's good for me.
>
> "I do want to have a second piece of pie because it tastes good. Sometimes, I do want to have hot, sweaty sex at night and again in the morning because it tastes good. I want to run to the roller coaster at Disneyland with the rest of the nine-year-old boys.
>
> "But I can't. The pie is bad for my weight and cholesterol. Pursuit of the morning sex will disturb my exhausted, sleeping spouse and negatively affect my marital love. The other parents at Disneyland will think I'm weird.

"We all know what moderation, control, and discipline really means. It means I don't get to have what I want. I get to watch other people have what I want and seem to get away with it. I get to convince myself that raw vegetables taste as good as a Krispy Kreme® doughnut. I don't just delay my gratification, frequently I don't get my gratification.

I know I need to be somewhat moderate, disciplined, and controlled to live effectively and for a long time, both of which I want. But what about passion, the juice of life? I love being passionate. Does passion have room for control and moderation or does it eat them? Does sensual, hedonistic pleasure have to wear the belt of moderation? I don't think so.

"The wonder of new romance is reflected in doing things over the top; being infatuated and going with it through cards and letters and three-hour phone calls and getting into work late and tired. Real passion for something makes everything else seem like white noise and static. Passion almost demands that other things be put aside so that you can be excessive.

"For a year, I wrote my first book, *Stepping Stones: 10 Steps to Seizing Passion and Purpose* between 9:00 p.m. and 2:00 a.m. every day and on weekends, feeling possessed with a needful sense of urgency to write. I'm ashamed to admit that it was a great experience even though I didn't spend as much time with my family.

"As I look back, I think the times I've been happiest in my life, I have been obsessed and passionate about something: school, a woman, building my career, exercise, etc. At those times, I was almost never moderate. I didn't necessarily feel out of control, but I was definitely consumed by my passion. It was effortful to pull myself away for long periods.

"Is passion and purpose something you have to balance? Or does being passionate help you with your purpose and vice versa? If you try to balance passion and mature, effective living, are you cheating yourself out of both? Can you hurl yourself into a pleasurable moment and be moderate? I don't know.

"I need to go now. My spinach salad and diet 7-Up are getting warm."

Moderating and Modifying Your Enjoyable Activities

Moderating and modifying enjoyable activities is difficult and requires a delicate balance between maintaining enjoyment and just going through the motions. Bill was a patient who had been coaching Little League baseball for years even after his son was too old to play. Bill had found it nearly impossible to coach after he injured his right arm.

He described the joy he got from coaching and demonstrating the proper playing techniques to the players. We agreed that he would try to modify his coaching style so that he did not have to demonstrate things, like how to field a ground ball or hit to the opposite field. He found that not only did he no longer enjoy coaching, but also that coaching this way was a constant reminder of what he had lost. He made the decision to stop coaching and ceased all involvement in Little League administration. Ultimately, I think this was a tragic but perfectly healthy choice for Bill.

The Power in Finding New and Pleasurable Activities

You probably have many enjoyable activities that you either cannot modify or if modified you would not enjoy them enough to want to continue with them. So, what then? You must find other pleasurable activities that are within your physical comfort zone. It is possible that these new activities will be as enjoyable as or more so than the old ones, although it is more likely that you selected the previous activities because they were the most intrinsically enjoyable. Regardless, you need to bring new enjoyable activities into your life. This is an example of what happens when people stop putting their lives on hold and begin to accept pain and courageously move forward with their lives. You stop waiting to have fun until you feel better.

HOW TO DEVELOP A PLEASURE PYRAMID TO HAVE MORE FUN

You can integrate into your Personal Pain Paradigm a hierarchy of enjoyable activities called a Pleasure Pyramid. You can be creative and plan to explore several new activities. I ask my patients to work on building a list of ten to thirty activities that could be fun for them to do and that are within their physical limits. Some activities will be quiet fun, hopefully some are loudly enjoyable, but at a minimum, you can still have fun. You should spend time thinking about this list and explore various options. As you develop your Pleasure Pyramid, place these new activities in hierarchical order from most to least enjoyable.

Take a long look at the calendar or weekend section of several local newspapers. You can find hundreds of local events each week, many of which are free or nearly so if your finances are tight. You can look at the myriad of city or county papers or magazines like the Penny Saver. You can look in the adult education section of your local community college's course catalog for classes that might be interesting and fun to take, possibly with an eye toward starting a new hobby.

Arts, crafts, and hobbies are wonderful distractions from pain that can be fun and provide a sense of accomplishment, too. You can get back in touch with a previous activity that you dropped. You can go to craft stores or hobby shops, get some ideas, and check out the incredible supplies that are available for various activities. You can go on the Internet and look up *fun things to do.* When this book was written, Yahoo listed 34 million web sites and Google listed 21 million websites describing fun things to do. You could also join several Internet groups. My patient, Ron, lives to play an Internet golf game with other Internet golfers. Ted loves to play an Internet fantasy, adventure game called World of Warcraft. All of these activities could be placed on your Pleasure Pyramid.

You might find enjoyable activities that are just outside your physical limitations even with moderation or modification. You could put a few of these on a separate list and use them as motivation to adhere to your global plan for self-management. As you become better conditioned and more able to do things, you can slowly begin to engage in more challenging and pleasurable activities. This is a great way to reward yourself for persevering with self-management.

We know that chronic pain produces limitations that can severely affect your ability to engage in pleasurable activities. We learned that lack of fun can lead to depression. One of the major symptoms of depression is anhedonia, literally meaning without pleasure. When people are severely depressed, the whole world can seem gray and joyless. This means that even when you engage in previously enjoyable activities within your physical limits, you may not experience joy from them anymore. You are just going through the motions.

In the chapter on pain behaviors, we discussed the importance of acting "as if" you do not have pain where appropriate. In other contexts, you may act as if you like the person to whom you are talking; as if the meal tastes good; or as if you like your job or boss. We all do this. It's necessary sometimes to act this way to avoid offending someone, to be civil, and to continue supporting ourselves or to remain employed. Such is the business of life.

So, too, is the business of pain and depression. You should continue to engage in activities that used to be fun even if they no longer are, as long as they are within your limits. If you do not, your depression will worsen and you will become less active and more withdrawn. If you practice what you are learning in this book, and continue to participate in previously enjoyable activities, they will become fun again. This may happen slowly and incrementally, but it will happen.

Your Pleasure Pyramid becomes a reminder of fun and a gateway to pleasurable activity. It's easy to become so wrapped up in the daily hassles and chores of life that you forget to have fun. When you hurt, it becomes even less natural to perform enjoyable activities. The Pleasure Pyramid is like an old friend quietly waiting to have a good time with you.

Spend a few minutes a week with your pyramid and incorporate a few of the items into your short, medium, and long-term goals. Be mindful of new possibilities for fun. My patient, Peter, builds free-flying, gasoline-powered, model airplanes with which he enters contests on weekends. Each flight, he follows his plane on a mountain bike to retrieve it when it lands. How cool is that?

When you socialize, find out what other people do for fun. Add new items to your Pleasure Pyramid whenever you can, and try to do something pleasurable at least weekly. You deserve to have fun.

I can maintain enjoyable activities even with chronic pain

Insight—I understand the benefits of pleasurable activity even though I hurt.
Commitment—I am committed to having more fun and combating depression.
Action—I will develop a Pleasure Pyramid and add to it over the years.
Now—Right now, I can think of one activity within my limits that's fun, and that is: _____

_____

_____

19

How to Be Productive and Maintain Life Purpose

Chronic pain inevitably decreases your productivity. It places physical limitations on you. It decreases your ability to think, attend, concentrate, and solve problems. You are less patient and more irritable. Your social skills decrease. Chronic pain affects people across all realms including physical, relational, mental, emotional, and spiritual. In almost every way, people in pain are aware that they are less effective and productive. This devolution tends to be greater as pain increases. These comments are not meant to make you feel worse about yourself but to acknowledge one aspect of the changing you.

WHY IS PRODUCTIVE ACTIVITY IMPORTANT WITH CHRONIC PAIN?

Productive activity is the central avenue through which people bring meaning and purpose into their lives. Purely physical, pleasurable, and social activities are important but seem mainly to provide a background for what gives life real meaning. Productive actions are those that produce something, whether tangible or not. They are behaviors that accomplish a goal or contribute in a positive way to self, family, community, or society.

Productive activities may be some combination of physical, social, or pleasurable activities. Examples include cleaning your house, talking to your child about right and wrong, picking up litter, planning your retirement, finishing your tax return, or putting a few dollars in the church basket. The key is that you can feel good about what you have done because, in some small way, you have made yourself or the world a better place.

Gainful employment is the most obvious example of productive activity and usually involves at least a little physical and social activity. Chronic pain can severely affect your ability to get things done and gainful employment may be difficult at best. In *Stepping Stones: 10 Steps to Seizing Passion and Purpose,* I stated, "Work...(is) based upon your ability to produce stuff, lots of stuff, and quickly. Work is stressful. That's why you get paid for it. Nobody at work has to be concerned about your feelings, needs, or goals. You're being paid. Stress and dysfunction increase geometrically and whatever dark craziness lurks inside your personality, it is likely to come out under the stress of work. Yet, your chosen career and your effectiveness become a major part of your identity."

Thus, chronic pain can change your fundamental perception of who you are, i.e., your self-identity. More than any other complaint, my patients will say, "I don't know who I am any more. I used to have goals and achieve them. I used to work hard and feel good about it. I used to be constantly in motion doing things. I have become a new person. I don't know who this person is; but I don't think I like em' very much."

Worse than the suffering from decreased physical, pleasurable, or social activity, many people with chronic pain complain of a lack of being productive, of not feeling valuable anymore, or of not having a sense of purpose. This happens most often when the person was gainfully employed at the onset of the pain problem but is no longer.

STRATEGIES FOR MAINTAINING EMPLOYMENT WITH CHRONIC PAIN

If you have chronic pain, maintaining your employment may be one of your most important tasks. You are not just continuing to work; you are sustaining your basic sense of identity as a worker, a productive human being contributing in some way to society. Because work is mentally and physically stressful, however, it probably increases your pain.

Most of my patients who are working full time and take one to four weeks off to focus on their Personal Pain Paradigm program report a significant decrease in pain during this break. They may experience a new awareness of how much their work had been increasing their pain throughout the day, and decisions must be made about modifying their job to better manage their pain.

Work-related decisions are complicated because they tap into your basic sense of meaning and purpose. Work structures your day and compels distraction from pain precisely because it is stressful, hectic, and no one has to care about the fact that you hurt. However, over 80 percent of people in pain report increased pain as their day progresses anyway, regardless of their work status.

If you stop working, structure goes out the window and can leave you trapped in the paralysis of "I do what I can." I have observed hundreds of patients make a fully informed, apparently healthy decision to quit work, but over the next several years spiral down into depression, inactivity, and obsessing about pain, disability, and medical providers. They become the people they used to frown on in pain class. The immediate benefits of quitting work may be decreased pain, but the long-term costs may be increased pain and suffering. This is quite a quandary with certainty available only from hindsight.

Modifying Your Work Environment and Schedule

You may need to modify your employment to manage pain more effectively. This could mean changing your chair, desk, or other equipment to make your workspace more ergonomic. It could mean trying to change your hours or days. I treat patients whose working schedules use flextime, e.g., four, ten-hour days, and they choose their day off. Almost everyone picks Friday, whereas a few take Mondays off. Nevertheless, if you are committed to good pacing and limit setting, you are probably better off selecting Wednesdays, so you are never more than two days away from a break.

Most of my patients will say that they give 110 percent effort toward their work. They perceive themselves as working much harder than their co-workers. It is widely known that among people who are injured at work, a disproportionate number are injured after working eight hours in a day or forty hours in a week. Mostly, these people are the "gunners," the motivated ones doing the lion's share of the work in the office or the shop. This contrasts sharply with the popular perception of worker's compensation patients as lazy workers "scamming the system."

Redefining Your Sense of Identity

For workers accustomed to giving 110 percent, hard work becomes incorporated into their basic sense of identity. Pride, self-esteem, and life purpose meld into the belief that "I am a hard worker." Yet, you may need to moderate or decrease the intensity or quantity of your work. You may need to restrict yourself to only forty hours per week and allow yourself to be comfortable with the perception that you are now only an average worker. Or let yourself realize that, although you feel substandard, it is only because your standards for your performance are so high.

Your pride and self-esteem can stem from the fact that you are still a good worker and are managing a level of pain greater than any of your colleagues. It may well be that if you continued to work sixty hours per week at 110 percent effort; you would end up working zero hours weekly at 0 percent effort.

Unfortunately, no matter how well you organize your work setting and habits, you may not be capable of maintaining your current job on a full-time basis. You may need to request a part-time schedule, at least on a temporary basis, to give yourself more time for your self-management. I realize that there may be some real world issues of finances or fringe benefits that can make this decision a difficult one, but part-time work might be necessary. Full-time work combined with family demands places severe limits on how much time you can devote to exercise and self-management.

The physical and mental demands of your job might be so great that you cannot function adequately even part time. You might need to quit and find other work that is less demanding. This can be an excruciating decision as the new job would probably pay less, be less prestigious, and be less intrinsically satisfying. You might believe that you could not find other work or that the work would pay so little or be so unpleasant that it would not be worth the effort. Or, perhaps you are skeptical because you have tried other jobs, and were unable to succeed at them.

THE FOUR PATHS TO MEANING AND PURPOSE WITHOUT EMPLOYMENT

One way or another, you may find yourself unemployed, unstructured, and bored, at least when you are not totally consumed by a severe pain episode. How do you find meaning and purpose when you are not gainfully employed? How can you feel valuable and do more than just keep busy? First, you might realize that stay-at-home moms have been dealing with this issue for millennia. It is not new or specific to you. It just feels weird and bad. Then you realize that paid work is only the most obvious example of productive activity. Wages represent a societal recognition that what you have done that day or week has value. However, very important, productive work is often unpaid which can mean unrecognized. You can perform many unpaid activities that might be more valuable and provide an even greater sense of purpose.

In *Stepping Stones: 10 Steps to Seizing Passion and Purpose,* I observed that people tend to find meaning and purpose through four interdependent paths:

- Personal happiness

- Improving the welfare of others

- Contributing to the planet itself

- Glorifying your god(dess).

People in pain are often confronted with these issues for the first time because of the pain-related changes in their lives.

Personal Happiness through Self-Awareness, Integrity, and the Mastery Map

The first path toward meaning is personal happiness. This path includes self-awareness, integrity, and mastery of life tasks. You can consciously choose to enhance these three aspects of happiness.

Self-awareness involves increasing your understanding of yourself, especially your strengths and weaknesses. When you have chronic pain, you should emphasize awareness of your strengths, and the qualities that you still like about yourself. You may already spend too much time thinking about your weaknesses, although, you may work to maintain a more realistic perception of your weaknesses. For instance, you are not a bad father because you cannot play catch with your son. Becoming more self-aware also means recognizing and accepting the changing you, not the way you were or want to be, but the way you are.

Having integrity means living your life according to your values and goals. Superficially, it is living according to common standards of social effectiveness and basic decency. Grossly aberrant behavior, like rape or murder, cannot reflect integrity no matter how messed up your values are. At a deeper level, integrity means basing your actions on those values that you believe are the most important to you. It means being willing to stand up for what you think is right or just. It requires courage, and the willingness to be loyal to an idea or a principle. True courage can be defined as integrity in action. Chronic pain cannot take away or reduce your integrity. In fact, you can even re-commit to acting in accordance with your values and beliefs.

Personal mastery can be severely challenged by chronic pain. You are highly likely to perceive yourself as less competent, independent, and in control of your life. Your mastery of basic life tasks probably decreases as your pain increases. Maintaining a sense of personal mastery may be the most important psychological task facing people with chronic pain, depression, and loss.

I developed the Mastery Map to help people increase their sense of mastery and self-esteem no matter what their physical condition. Your Mastery Map is a hierarchy of activities or goals that are difficult, scary, or otherwise challenging, but would be healthy, maturing, or self-actualizing if you did them. These tasks are not usually directly related to pain and so should be well within your physical limits. Accomplishing these tasks will create self-esteem and a sense of meaning that may have been damaged by pain and limitations.

The Mastery Map is meant to tap into your darker side, the idiosyncratic side, the bottomless pit where you put away little secrets or fears that you might not want anyone else to know. Put another way, these activities may get you where you live. They make you less effective and whole, less integrated. They are the boxes that you never open, the ones that clutter and obstruct your life's journey.

Maybe you dropped out of high school and never found the time to get your diploma or equivalency degree. Perhaps you are afraid to drive on the freeways. Maybe you have not undergone a routine dental, gynecologic, or breast exam in years. Maybe you have not filed taxes in several years. You might be avoiding confronting someone or putting off a necessary decision. Maybe you are afraid to look at your credit report or screen your phone calls because of collection agents. Perhaps you are avoiding some necessary chore like cleaning the garage. Maybe you always wanted to read a certain book or take a particular class. Perhaps you have been putting off learning to use a computer or surf that newfangled Internet. Maybe you want to be less verbally critical of your spouse. These are perfect issues to place on your Mastery Map.

The most powerful and poignant Mastery Map issue I can recall was a 63-year-old, African American patient raised in the rural south who tearfully confessed after pain class one day that he had never learned to read. He understood a few basic words and could recognize frequently used signs and traffic signals, but his reading was at about first grade level. He was considered illiterate. We found him an adult education class for beginning reading adults, but he dropped out of treatment with me soon after. However, a year later, he returned for a session and showed me he could read at a high school level. This time we both cried.

An example from my own life is a little less poignant. By nature, I tend to pay more attention to people than to things, and in my teens and early twenties, I had a very poor sense of direction. As a teenager, when I was driving outside of my familiar area, I would become lost rather frequently. When I went out with my friends, I often counted on them to navigate. This was not much more than an inconvenience, but it made me feel bad about myself. I decided to conquer this problem in three ways. First, I began keeping track of the direction in which I was traveling whenever I left the house regardless of who was driving. Second, I began studying maps whenever I left my familiar area. Third, when I was twenty-one, I began a job selling biomedical equipment throughout the Midwestern United States. On my sales trips, which were always by car and alone, I paid special attention to directions and forced myself to always know in what direction I was traveling and where the hotel and client were in relation to my location.

Within a couple years, I had successfully conquered my problem and I learned to navigate very quickly when I moved to Southern California. I challenged this problem long before I developed the concept of the Mastery Map. You have probably challenged or conquered weaknesses or fears similarly.

Over the next few months, think about tasks or goals that you might include in your Mastery Map. Place them in a hierarchical order from easiest to hardest based upon how challenging they are and how long they will take to accomplish. As you add items to your Mastery Map, you must develop a step-by-step plan for accomplishing each task. Long-term tasks or goals should be broken down into medium-and short-term goals. You should write down when and how you will accomplish each step. For time-consuming tasks, you should carve out a few hours per week to work on them. The items on this map probably should not be pain related, i.e., they should be well within your physical limits.

Your Mastery Map will take a lifetime to complete as you add new items and as old ones fall off once they are completed. Some items, like learning how to read, may require a longer term, steady commitment and remain on the map for years. Others, like reviewing your credit report, may be finished after the first time they are addressed.

Ultimately, the Mastery Map is a scientific approach that's geared not just toward meaning and purpose, but also toward self-esteem. Your map becomes part of the goal setting, planning, and structure within your Personal Pain Paradigm. Once an item is on the list, you need to be persevering. You will feel good about yourself as you work on the issues on your map. You will feel stronger and more capable knowing that you can trust yourself more. Pain makes people feel so weak and vulnerable. The Mastery Map helps you reclaim your power, passion, and purpose.

Meaning and Purpose through Altruism

Improving yourself is important but many people feel a special joy and value mostly when they help others. Directing your productive efforts toward helping others can be intensely meaningful. You might also have existing activities that you would like to extend or expand. Perhaps you volunteer at church or temple and you might want to do more of that. You might volunteer at a local hospital or become a mentor or Big Brother or Sister. Perhaps you simply make a commitment to spending more time with your family while being more aware of your role as a family educator and listener. You could set up or participate in a support group on the Internet for people in pain. Frequently, the value of a life is not in the few big things, but in the million little things that you do to enrich the lives of your family, friends, and community. You may long for "larger than life," concrete examples of your positive influence on others, but your real value may lie in all the little things you do along the way.

I remember a patient who told me about an experience that occurred at his mother's funeral. She had been a quiet, loving woman, a schoolteacher who never seemed too busy to help others. He said there were over a thousand people at her service, the largest funeral in the city's history. It took hours for those gathered to finish the loving tributes for that wonderful woman who had lived with chronic pain since her late teens.

Changing what you do can be important with chronic pain, but changing how you perceive yourself may be just as important.

Love of Nature Can Transcend Pain

The meaning of transcending yourself or other people can be found in literally "making the world a better place." This includes living in harmony with nature. Over the course of a lifetime, you will generate tons of garbage and pollution, but you can minimize this destructiveness and even become one of earth's assets. You can participate actively in recycling programs. You can minimize use of non-organic chemicals and sprays. You can pick up litter on a regular basis and encourage others to do so. You can conserve water and electricity. You can learn about our natural resources and get involved by joining environmental groups and donating time or money. You can really make a difference and feel good about it.

Spirituality Can Integrate and Comfort a Painful Life

Finally, people with chronic pain can create meaning and purpose through their spirituality and productively spiritual behaviors. For some people it means recommitting to their God(dess). For others, it may be as simple as attending church or temple more regularly. It may mean joining a religious study group. You might volunteer time in your church or in charitable activities of your temple or mosque. You might want to read various pain books that combine spirituality and pain management like Timothy Hansel's, *You Gotta Keep Dancing*. Recent research suggests that people who use spirituality in a moderate way to cope with pain actually cope better than those who are not spiritual at all or are too fervently religious. Food for thought.

A spiritually loving approach to life envelops and supports you. It celebrates and exults in the good times and provides comfort through the bad times. You can feel more centered and less isolated through your spirituality even if you hurt. Prayer can be a powerful force in your life. But it should be in addition to, and not in place of, all the other things you can do to help yourself. Even God would agree, "Sometimes you just need to jump out of the way of the truck."

I can be productive and feel purposeful even with chronic pain

Insight—I understand the four paths to meaning and purpose: self, others, planet, God(dess).
Commitment—I am committed to organizing my goals across the four paths.
Action—I will develop a Mastery Map and begin accomplishing the items on it.
Now—Right now, I can think of one scary thing I wish I didn't avoid and it is:

_____

_____

20

How to Change Pain-related Thoughts and Be Less Miserable

Pain does not make you feel any particular emotion. The way you think about your pain does. Pain does not make you feel angry, sad, scared, guilty, or ashamed. The immediate thought you have about your pain determines which of the thousands of possible negative emotions you will experience.

In Chapter 6, we discussed the fact that pain was defined as an unpleasant physical and emotional experience, and that pain was almost never purely physical or emotional, but fluctuates on a continuum between the two. The international change in the definition of pain was driven in part by the realization that the experience of chronic pain tended to be associated with much more suffering. It is a more unpleasant experience than acute pain. Since acute and chronic pain are not the same thing, the negative thoughts and feelings associated with chronic pain are not just quantitatively different from those related to acute pain. They are qualitatively different. You do not just suffer more with chronic pain but in a different way.

Albert Ellis pioneered the field of Rational Emotive Therapy within what was referred to as the third wave of psychology. Sigmund Freud championed the first wave at the turn of the twentieth century in which he believed that behavior and emotions were caused by drives or instincts especially sexual and productive ones. B.F. Skinner championed the behavioral conditioning model in which behaviors and emotions were considered to be driven by stimulus-response connections. The third wave loosely championed by Albert Ellis, Albert Bandura, and Abraham Maslow conceived of emotions and behaviors driven mainly by the meaning that was attached to the events in our lives. This made instinctual urges and stimulus-response connections less central to human psychology.

195

How Thoughts Affect Feelings and Behaviors

Ellis developed the A-B-C-D model of human activity in which an antecedent event (A) results in a consequent emotion (C) because of an intervening belief or thought (B). Then people engage in a decisional behavior (D). This model is written as $A+B=C \rightrightarrows D$. The modern definition of pain as an unpleasant physical and emotional experience is consistent with the fact that we give pain meaning, and that meaning largely determines our feelings about our pain, and what we subsequently do about it.

Jane had chest pain that was often excruciating. We can call her sensation of pain the antecedent event (A). This pain terrified her. Fear would be the consequent emotion (C). The pain terrified her because she interpreted it to mean that she was having a heart attack and dying, a thought, or belief (B). The antecedent pain combined with the belief that she was dying produced the consequent terror. Natural fluctuations in her pain, especially pain increases, led her to believe that death was imminent, which caused increased fear, and she often decided (D) to go to the emergency room or call her doctor at all hours. Our primary task was to change her belief in the meaning of her pain especially the phasic increases in her pain. She learned that her chest pain varied naturally, like all chronic pain, and that she would likely continue to have periods of severe pain. She learned that these episodes did not mean that she was dying, and that her increased pain was not associated with increased injury. We also taught her relaxation exercises and a range of other self-management techniques. She learned to cope without medical professionals and stopped pursuing emergency medical treatment during severe pain episodes.

Distorted Thoughts that Make Us Miserable

Ellis and subsequent theorists in cognitive behavioral psychology developed a list of types or patterns of thoughts or beliefs that make us more miserable than we have to be because they are distorted or unhealthy in some way. David Burns and his colleagues expanded this notion to include a list of Automatic Negative Thoughts (ANTs) that create or exaggerate negative emotions. There are as many different lists as there are theorists out there but a few seem especially applicable to pain and associated suffering. Understanding ANTs and other cognitive distortions is one of your most powerful weapons against pain.

Polarized Thinking

The most important distorted negative thought related to pain is called polarized, black and white, or all-or-none thinking. When you think about an event in a polarized manner, you may perceive it as all good or all bad and respond with extremely negative emotions based upon all bad. This is one of the two most common cognitive distortions for people in pain.

When patients say that their pain is a level 100 on a scale of 0-100 and they demonstrate minimal pain behavior and laugh much of the time, they are probably not accurate in their pain assessment. This does not mean that they are lying. They may simply be saying, "Look doc, my pain is terrible so I'm calling it a 100. When y'all get rid of it, I'll call it a zero." When patients say that their pain does not vary at all during a typical day, this too is not accurate, but more likely reflective of the same polarized thinking, not actual lying.

The problem with polarized thinking is that it distorts reality and makes you much more miserable, much more angry, anxious, sad, or guilty than you would be otherwise. Polarized thinking is actually hardwired at birth. Infants are born with their senses full on and the ability to distinguish between pleasure and pain. Their emotional reactions reflect the fact that they perceive the world in a very all-or-none way. They are not "a little unhappy" about anything. They seem to be content, sleeping, or screaming bloody murder.

As infants get older, they begin to distinguish among a variety of all-or-none, or black and white sensations like hungry-full, wet-dry, and cold-warm. As they mature through childhood, they learn that most life events are on a continuum, various shades of gray in-between black and white. They can be a little hungry and learn that if they wait a few minutes they will still get fed even if they do not cry.

Indeed, effective living requires maneuvering within the shades of gray between black and white. We all need to learn that mothers do not have to be all good all the time. You do not have to be perfect. Happiness is often found in "good enough," and not in perfection. You can realize that mild pain is a lot better than severe pain.

We have a natural tendency to perceive the world in a relatively polarized way because it is easier and simpler to do so. It is hard work to make the fine discriminations necessary when you choose to see events or choices on a continuum. It is much easier to base your actions on an all-or-none perception. For instance, infatuation is that glorious "all good" stage in a relationship when you see your partner as almost all good and you can throw yourself full throttle into the relationship with minimal hesitancy. It becomes much more complicated when you are forcibly confronted over time with the "bad" parts, and must decide if the good outweighs the bad, or if your partner is good enough.

In a given situation, polarized thinking allows for easier decisional behaviors even though it makes you more intensely emotional. In what types of situations are you most highly motivated to see an event in an all-or-none way? When you are faced with a decision that has an all-or-none outcome, you may tend to perceive your selected choice as all good. When you decide to buy a particular car, you find yourself noticing all the wonderful things about it while ignoring all the bad things, similar to what we do early in relationships.

When you are in a hurry, you may see things in an all-or-none way because you do not have the time or desire to make fine discriminations. When you are tired, you may not have the energy to make fine discriminations. When you are emotionally stressed or upset, you are less interested in making fine discriminations.

Sometimes when I am in a hurry, tired, and stressed, I find myself dividing human beings into two groups, those who make my life easier and those who make my life harder. It does not matter much if it's a little easier, or a little harder, or a lot. I may respond emotionally as if it's a lot, or so my wife tells me.

People with chronic pain tend to engage in polarized thinking more than those who do not have chronic pain, because they are usually tired due to sleep deprivation, and trying to manage their pain. They are stressed almost continually because of pain, and they may constantly feel rushed as they try to accomplish tasks with a body that is functioning much more slowly than it once did.

Life is so effortful when you have chronic pain that you will leap to take shortcuts that make it seem easier, like seeing people, pain, and events in a polarized way. In the short run, your decisions are easier, but you are made more miserable. You suffer more in the end because of your polarized thinking.

In the specific case of perceiving pain itself in an all-or-none way, you cannot meaningfully judge the efficacy of medical treatments that affect your pain by only a little or appreciate small steps in recovery. Hope and optimism with pain are predicated on being able to appreciate and hang on to baby steps in improvement. Evaluate your thought processes and try to notice when you are engaging in polarized thinking. Take a few moments to identify the gray area in any given situation.

Musterbation

Another important cognitive distortion for people in pain is called the "musts" or the "shoulds." People carry around with them thousands of beliefs, many of them based on childhood experiences, about how the world works and should work. They know how they believe they should behave and how the people around them should behave. We make ourselves miserable when we violate our own shoulds or when other people do. We feel more angry, sad, guilty, ashamed, or afraid than we would otherwise.

Chronic pain places limits on our behavior and affects pleasurable, social, and productive activity. These changes conflict with many of our shoulds and make us miserable. You may get angry because you believe that you should not hurt so much and that, if you do, the medical system has failed. You may feel frustrated and lonely if you believe that as long as you are in pain, i.e., sick, your support system should rally around your flagpole. You may feel guilty if you believe that you should work hard and that if you are not working hard then you are a lazy slug.

You may feel ashamed if you believe that you should always be nice or be in a good mood, which is nearly impossible when you have chronic pain. You may believe that people should like you, but know that you are not as likable when your pain is severe. You may be wracked with guilt about not spending as much time with your spouse, children, or extended family as you think you should because you hurt so much.

If the healthy enemy of perfection is "good enough" then the healthy enemy of should is "want to." Most of the shoulds are not societally mandated standards of morality, like "I should not steal or kill," but internalized perceptions of the kind of person you want to be or the kind of society you would like to have. The shoulds related to being nice, working hard, or spending more time with your family are not black and white moral issues with an absolute standard, but rather, a style of living that you want to maintain.

You place intense pressure on yourself by believing that you should perform a behavior rather than simply wanting to perform it. This pressure does increase the likelihood that you will perform the behavior. However, the shoulds also create an artificially rigid performance standard and make you unnecessarily miserable when you do not live up to them.

Some cognitive distortions exaggerate naturally occurring emotions, and some, like the shoulds, inevitably produce a particular emotion. When you do not live up to your shoulds, you will tend to feel guilty. When other people do not live up to your shoulds, you will tend to feel angry.

The Blaming Syndrome

Blaming is another cognitive distortion that seems to result from chronic pain. Initially, people in pain feel guilty and sad about all the activities they can no longer perform. But, as your activities become restricted and your pain does not go away, you may find yourself increasingly blaming others for your misery, most often when they do not live up to your shoulds.

When you hurt, marital and familial conflict is almost inevitable as your spouse begins to take over your previous responsibilities or they simply do not get done. You will probably begin blaming your spouse for things with the perception that your spouse is not being supportive enough, or caring enough and should be. Over time, it may feel that the reason you are miserable so often is due to how your spouse responds to your pain.

You need to remember that you are responsible for how you feel, since it is the way you think about events that creates your feelings, not specifically what is happening. If your spouse is irritated or frustrated with you, that frustration does not have to make you feel anything. You choose how you will feel by choosing how you think about it. Moreover, you can choose not to feel angry, bitter, or hurt. Ultimately, you are fully responsible for what you think, feel, and do.

Internal and External Control Fallacies

The shoulds and blaming behaviors blend into the next two pain-related cognitive distortions—the internal and external control fallacies. The internal control fallacy is the cognitive behavioral term for thoughts and actions that are commonly called codependent. Here you believe that you are responsible for the happiness or distress of another person even when you have not caused it or do not have any control over it.

If you are lying on the couch when your spouse comes home (his event A) and he thinks you should not be (his belief B), he may be angry with you (his consequent emotion C) and start complaining about you lying down (his decisional behavior D). His complaining is your event (A) and you may believe that you are at fault for his anger (your belief B) which produces guilty feelings in you (your consequent emotion C) and leads you to apologize and withdraw to your bedroom (your decisional D). With the internal control fallacy, you take responsibility for another person's thoughts, feelings, or behaviors, which usually leads to guilt and self-recrimination. Any time you take full responsibility for another person's thoughts, feelings, or actions, you are guilty of the internal control fallacy.

The external control fallacy is the logical flip side of the internal control fallacy. If you believe that you are to blame for what other people think, feel, or do, you may give yourself permission to blame other people or events for what you think, feel, and do. This allows you to deny responsibility for your own thoughts, feelings, and behaviors perceiving them as completely out of your control. This style of distorted thinking is classically seen in physically abusive men who comment "I wouldn't have hit the b**** if she hadn't burned the dinner. She knows that pushes my buttons." The man denies any responsibility for his role in the abuse and blames her because she knows her actions will push his button, and once his button is pushed, he cannot be held accountable.

Many people in pain maintain an external control fallacy over pain in general. They feel helpless and victimized in the belief that their pain is almost entirely out of their control. Their interactions with their pain doctors can become increasingly desperate and childlike. If you believe that your doctor holds the only keys to the doors of pain relief, you will feel more scared and needy, which may lead to impulsive decisional behaviors like pleading for a pain shot or demanding more narcotics.

In this context, I have commented to physicians and patients alike that the typical emergency room (E.R.) visit for severe chronic pain is more a psychological emergency than a medical one. This is not to say that severe pain is not real, but more that the E.R. visit is born of fear—that the severe pain will not go away; that the severe pain is reflective of a new problem; or of the belief that the E.R. doctors can and should be able to make the pain go away and quickly.

Patients are often outraged when they are forced to wait six hours in the E.R., compelled to undergo diagnostic tests when all they want is pain relief, or are given weak pain medicine in the form of Toradol injections or Vicodin. While the external control fallacy drives them to the E.R., once there, the shoulds and blaming distortions drive their dissatisfaction with the treatment received. Many E.R. doctors do not believe it is their role to manage severe pain episodes in the absence of an acute injury.

Catastrophizing

Catastrophizing is a common cognitive distortion that refers to thinking about an event in terms of the worst possible outcome and then responding emotionally not to the event itself, but to the worst possible outcome. Pain and the associated misfortunes seem to propel nasty future thoughts, including potential death, increased injury, financial ruin, or relational destruction.

If you have a herniated disc in your neck that is causing pain in your right arm and months or years later develop pain in your left arm, the most likely explanation is that you have been compensating and overusing the left arm, which has caused muscle soreness, or some type of inflammation. However, if you obsess about other more terrible things (B) that could be causing the left arm pain (A), your anxiety and fear (C) will escalate indefinitely and you may engage in increasingly desperate and unhealthy behaviors (D) as a result. The more pain and distress you experience, and the more preoccupied you are with your pain, the more time you will probably spend catastrophizing and the more miserable you will be.

Personalization

The final pain-related type of cognitive distortion is called personalization. In this pattern of thought, you find yourself thinking about an event that does not really involve you as if it did, and feel worse about yourself or engage in unhealthy behavior. You can personalize all of the characteristics of other people that you want or used to have before pain.

Another person (event A) may be seen as richer, better looking, thinner, happier, or having less pain than you (belief B) which makes you feel worse about yourself (emotion C). You can personalize all the activities that other people can do that you used to be able to perform and feel miserable about yourself as a result. Instead of enjoying watching a baseball game, you may focus on how much you enjoyed playing baseball before your pain began. This will make you unhappy and bring down your self-esteem.

Over the years, my pain classes have enjoyed an example of my own personalization. My wife came home from work one day and was being distant, quiet, and vaguely irritable toward me. I assumed that she was upset with me. Naturally, I adopted the attitude that the best defense is a strong offense and I attacked her verbally. I explained that I had not done anything wrong, that I was not responsible for her being upset, and that I did not deserve her anger. She looked at me for what seemed like an eternity and then said, "Honey, not everything in my life is about you." I went from being 6' 2" tall to being 2" tall in about a second. Sorry, dear.

I can change my thoughts and be less miserable

Insight—I understand the A-B-C-D model of thoughts, feelings, and behaviors.
Commitment—I am committed to minimizing my use of cognitive distortions.
Action—I will be more aware of my thought patterns and battle distortions on land and sea.
Now—Right now, I can think of one distorted thought I engage in fairly often and that is:_____

_____

_____

21

How to Improve Your Attention, Concentration, and Memory

Moderate to severe chronic pain affects your ability to perform mental tasks. Neuropsychological testing on people in pain consistently demonstrates deficits in attention, concentration, short and long-term memory, problem-solving, decision-making, learning, and organization. More than 90 percent of the patients I have treated have acknowledged that mental tasks were more difficult with pain. The worse the pain, the more difficult it is to think effectively.

PAIN IS DISTRACTING

Pain is a powerful distraction from conducting the daily business of life. Attention is defined simply as turning your conscious awareness, senses, and thoughts toward something. Pain demands your attention in a manner similar to a screaming baby, freezing rain on your skin, or a horrific accident at the side of the road. It is possible to focus on other things but it takes increased effort to deliberately ignore the white elephant in the living room. This is further complicated by the fact that in a typical day you must pay attention to thousands of stimuli, often in rapid succession, and make decisions about the priority of the stimuli competing for your attention. This is tough when you hurt like hell.

Concentration is defined as longer-term attention on a single stimuli or task. To concentrate is to consciously maintain attention and persevere with it over time. While attention is difficult with pain, concentration is much harder since it requires much more effort. You have to concentrate to drive a car, play a video, or interpret a map. Concentration taxes the limited resources of someone in pain even more. It can fly in the face of effective pacing and limit setting. Serious concentration can eventually increase muscle-based pain or produce other pain, e.g., headaches or pains in weak body parts that do not normally hurt.

Short-term memory means remembering something for a few minutes. It is remembering a phone number you received from the operator long enough to dial the number or remembering where you just set your coffee mug. These tasks require that you transfer information (objects) to which you have attended into short-term memory storage. The worse you are attending and concentrating, the less successful you will be with this transfer.

The more stimuli or distractions that occur in your environment during and immediately after the transfer from attention to short-term memory, the less you will remember in the short term. For instance, if someone is giving you information over your cell phone while you are driving, and immediately afterward you witness an accident, it will be difficult to remember what the person on the phone said because the accident interferes with the transfer from attention to short-term memory.

The worst memory concerns voiced by people in pain are in situations that require incidental memory. With the above examples, memory for a phone number you just received from the operator is active, intentional memory. You know you need to remember this information for a little while. On the other hand, memory for where you put your coffee mug is incidental to the business of life. You are probably not consciously thinking, "Boy I hope I remember where I put this."

Most of us can remember most of these things during the course of a normal day when we are feeling and functioning pretty well. But, when you are in pain, sleep-deprived, depressed, or stressed out, you are far more likely not to remember these incidental events. It does not mean that you are crazy or losing it. It just means that you are struggling with severe stresses.

ASSESSING YOUR MENTAL PERFORMANCE

Problem solving and decision-making are also impaired by chronic pain. These are considered higher order brain functions as compared to attention, concentration, and memory. These tasks involve analysis or figuring something out. You need to simultaneously keep multiple ideas accessible in short-term memory. You have to integrate old information with new information and must prioritize the relative value or importance of each. These tasks are performed more effectively in a relatively stress-free environment.

You are confronted with decisions and problems thousands of times each day, many of which you resolve so quickly that they remain below your conscious awareness. Analysis that is more complicated will require at least some of your conscious awareness or attention.

If you are trying to decide whether to stay with your current pain doctor or find another one, you are confronted with a complicated problem that has many different perspectives with a diverse matrix of advantages and disadvantages. The more you hurt, the less well you manage the concentration, short-term memory, and analysis required to solve the problem and the less energy you have to devote to the effort. You are likely to default and go with the status quo of your current doctor because it is less effortful all around.

Chronic pain is never experienced in isolation and the deficits in effective thinking due to pain are exacerbated by other factors. Sleep deprivation is almost ubiquitous with chronic pain as the vast majority of people with significant pain sleep fewer hours and less restfully when they do sleep. Many people with pain are also anxious or depressed which further compromises mental performance. Ninety-five percent of my patients take some type of medicine, any of which can impair mental performance. The classic daily medication regimen for pain patients includes a narcotic, muscle relaxant, anti-convulsant, anti-inflammatory, and sleeping agent, which in combination invariably affects mental performance at least a little.

How You Can Improve Mental Functioning in a Pain-Filled Life

Managing pain effectively also means managing the cognitive deficits caused by pain and associated sequelae. Patients complain frequently about their cognitive disruption but do little beyond bringing it to their doctor's attention. Some patients wonder if an additional medication will help. Some assume they just have to live with it, until their pain is decreased by their doctor. The truth is that there is a lot you can do to improve your mental functioning, including utilizing techniques we have already discussed. The issue is twofold. First, how can I improve my mental functioning? Second, how can I organize my environment so I do not have to function as well mentally?

Learn How to Structure Your Life

Structuring your life as much as possible improves your mental functioning and makes it easier to remember things. Arising and going to bed at the same time each day is helpful. Exercising at the same time each day is good. Setting up a schedule for physical, social, pleasurable, and productive activity is helpful. You need to have a basic routine that is consistent.

Focus on Increasing your Attention Span and Concentration Levels

Attention and concentration can be improved by being more mindful of things you want to remember and deliberately exerting more effort by observing things. The Sensory Training at Rest (STAR) and Sensory Training in Motion (STIM) techniques we discussed earlier are excellent ways of practicing attention and concentration, especially as you extend the time spent practicing them. You can practice concentrating by engaging in active, highly distracting activities, like video games, or talking to people for brief periods during which you fully commit to the effort necessary for intense concentration. Again, you can then extend the length of time you spend in these high demand activities.

Reviewing some strategies for short and long-term memory may be helpful. The most important is called rehearsal. If there is an event in your day that you want to remember, you pay special attention to it and repeat it immediately, several times if possible, and then repeat it a few more times in the next minutes or hours if you need to transfer it to long-term memory. The more often you repeat something, the better you will remember it. For instance, the best way to remember someone's name is to use it several times immediately upon meeting them and then again in conversation.

If you have several things to remember, you can try grouping them or using acronyms. A list of grocery items including bread, carrots, buns, sugar, celery, pork chops, hamburger, lipstick, eye shadow, flour, and eggs can be grouped into Vegetables, Breads, Meat, Cosmetics, and Ingredients, with each group having no more than three items. Then the acronym VBMCI is created from the first letter of each group, which might stand for Very Bad Memory Can Improve.

Ignore the Minor Things

Don't sweat the incidental memory lapses. You do not need to remember what you watched last night on television or what you had for breakfast. These things are not important and your life is minimally affected if you cannot remember them. Obsessing about not being able to remember them will make you more miserable and stressed, and will eventually make it even harder to remember things.

Keep in mind that people with genuinely severe cognitive deficits are often less aware of their deficits than are the people around them. People with mild mental compromise tend to be hyper-aware of small deficits that can feel larger than life. Additionally, people who are goal oriented, intelligent, highly productive, competent, or very busy tend to be more aware of small deficits, the kind that may take them from a superior level of functioning to an average level.

HOW TO ORGANIZE YOUR ENVIRONMENT TO OVERCOME MENTAL DYSFUNCTION

For the types of cognitive issues that stem from chronic pain, structuring your environment can be critical to lessen the impact of memory problems.

Create a Centralized System

In terms of incidental memory for keys, watch, wallet, etc, create a single place or two where you always put each item. As much as possible, organize your home so that frequently used and movable items have a single place where they are placed. Get in the habit of returning items to the storage place.

Walk through the various rooms in your home, especially bathrooms, family rooms, or den with an eye toward organization. Make sure you have cabinets for all your papers and labeled files available. The main goal in structure and organization is to create a system that does not rely on your internal memory to function efficiently. Then, when you have an item in your hand, expend the extra energy to put it back where it belongs.

Document Information in a Notebook Instead of Trying to Remember It

Perhaps the most important strategy for remembering things is to write them down. As difficult as daily function is for people in pain, it is nearly impossible for them to remember all of the information, appointments, issues, and questions associated with their various medical treatments. I encourage everyone with chronic pain to begin carrying around a planner or TAAP Journal to document information and to remember thoughts or ideas.

At the end of each day, see which tasks, appointments, or other relevant information are written down for the next day and then plan your activities accordingly. Any tasks that were not accomplished this day should be added to the next. It can also help if you keep a stack of sticky notes handy to transfer appointment dates and other time-sensitive information. Then just place the notes in strategic areas as reminders.

For many people in pain, writing things down on little notes and in a notebook is the single most important change they can make to help themselves function better mentally. Still, I would estimate that fewer than 50 percent of my patients maintain a notebook even after a course of behavioral treatment and repeated suggestions by me. Years may pass and they may continue to forget appointments, errands, medications, or self-management practice techniques. Many of these people continue to complain that they cannot remember anything and wonder what can be done to help them.

I can improve my mental functioning

Insight—I understand the impact of pain on attention, concentration, short-term memory, and problem solving.
Commitment—I am committed to improving my mental abilities.
Action—I will organize my environment better and write things down in a notebook.
Now—I think the best change I can make to improve my mental function is to:

_____

_____

_____

22

How to Manage Unhappy Emotions More Effectively

We have demonstrated that emotions are often produced by automatic thoughts and patterns of thought that may be consistent over time. It is nearly impossible to completely separate thoughts and feelings, or mental functioning and emotional functioning. Mental and emotional aspects of life are interdependent in the same way that sensations, thoughts, feelings, and behaviors are interdependent aspects of chronic pain. The mental and the emotional interact like one hand washing the other. However, we could note that mental functioning is more associated with how effectively we function, and emotional functioning is more associated with how satisfied we are with our functioning.

At the very least, emotions tend to occur at the end of a sequence of activities that include environmental events or sensations and thoughts. While thoughts may produce our feelings, our feelings give us tremendous insight into our thought patterns and exert tremendous influence over how we behave. Ultimately, pain is associated with negative emotions and managing pain successfully requires managing emotions successfully.

ACCURATELY LABELING FEELINGS HELPS YOU MANAGE THEM

Labeling your feelings accurately is the key to exercising control over them. You cannot change negative feelings if you do not know what they are. Unfortunately, people commonly do not identify or specify their negative emotions in various situations. When asked how you feel about an event, you may say, "It really upset me," or "It bothered me a little," or "I didn't like it much," or "I felt bad." These descriptions identify that you are feeling vaguely unhappy or dissatisfied, but do

210

not tell us why. Are you angry, sad, anxious, guilty, or ashamed? Do you feel any of the other hundred emotions in the English language? The most important task in managing your emotions is to clearly and consistently recognize and label the precise emotion you are experiencing in response to an event.

Identify Your True Feelings

There are three reasons why you may generalize your feelings into vague, non-descriptions. First, you may simply not recognize the feeling, perhaps because you have not experienced it before or because it is so mild. Second, you may be in the habit of not recognizing feelings because you are busy, or perpetually focused on other things. Third, you may deny or otherwise push your feelings out of consciousness, through what Freud referred to as defense mechanisms.

Regardless, healthy emotional management means giving yourself permission to recognize and label your feelings. When you find yourself saying or thinking that something bothers you, ask yourself what is the true underlying feeling? Test out a few of the global categories of emotions. Do I feel sad, angry, anxious, guilty, or ashamed?

COMMON PATTERNS OF FEELINGS THAT INCREASE SUFFERING FROM PAIN

If you are not sure what label to give your feeling, it may help to evaluate the situations or the thoughts that produced it. Certain patterns of thought reliably produce specific types of emotions. In *Stepping Stones: 10 Steps to Seizing Passion and Purpose*, I noted that you could infer feelings from thought patterns and vice versa as follows:

- Sad—Life is the pits because I lost something.

- Anxious—Life is the pits and it might get worse.

- Angry—Life is the pits and it's not fair or it's someone else's fault.

- Guilty—Life is the pits because of something I did and shouldn't have.

- Ashamed—Life is the pits because of something I did and shouldn't have and other people know it.

Many people tend toward feeling one emotion or another because they favor one of these thought patterns. You may tend toward sadness if you often think about all the things you have lost due to pain. You will tend to be anxious if you are forever imagining the worst possible outcomes of your pain problem. The more time you spend thinking about how unfair your pain condition is, or how other people are to blame, the more chronically angry you will become. The more time spent thinking about all the things you should be doing and are not, the guiltier you will feel. When you believe that other people notice the responsibilities that you are not fulfilling, the more often you will feel ashamed.

Assessing Emotional Patterns

It is helpful to be aware of stimuli that reliably produce a particular emotion. You can gain real information about yourself by assessing which events result in certain feelings. You may notice that some events produce feelings of anger, sadness, or anxiety without a clear reason. Perhaps a certain person or place makes you sad in the absence of any obvious cause. If this has occurred since you developed your pain, you can assume that something about that person or situation reminds you of your losses.

Gender differences in patterns of feelings are germane to people in pain. Men tend to be more motivated than women are by autonomy and individual achievement. They respond with anger to a wider variety of stimuli, in part because of frustration of achievement, and in part due to increased testosterone, which produces aggression. Anger is one of the more empowering emotions because it tends to make us feel stronger and less concerned about what others think. Males with chronic pain are somewhat more likely than females to be chronically angry. This affects their relationships negatively. It also increases pain through muscle tension and anger, driven by poor pacing and limit setting.

Women tend to be more motivated by affiliation than are men. Thus, they have more opportunities for perceived loss from chronic pain than men, which leads to sadness. They also tend to believe somewhat more intensely that they are letting family or friends down and so may feel guilt more often or more intensely. Events that men may respond to with anger, women may respond to with anxiety, which is also an energizing emotion, but not an empowering one. Anxiety increases chronic pain through muscle tension and autonomic arousal.

HONESTLY ASSESSING THE INTENSITY OF PAIN-RELATED FEELINGS

While managing emotions begins with accurately labeling them, you must also realistically assess the severity of your emotions. It is common, and at times healthy, to dampen your feelings to allow yourself to perform better. However, you may underestimate your feelings when you successfully mask them. You may think to yourself, "I feel irritated" when you are really feeling angry. You may think you are anxious when you are nearly terrified. The more you tend to squelch your feelings, the more you need to consider their true intensity. Your body's response to your feelings may be affected more by their actual severity and less by your dampened perception.

Some people tend to accentuate their feelings because of chronic severe stress and being taxed to the limits of their coping resources. Others employ cognitive distortions frequently. Still others have long-term character traits referred to as histrionic, obsessive-compulsive, narcissistic, or borderline. These people are driven by the matrix of their personality to intensify their original feelings. Unfortunately, their bodily responses and decision-making are likely to be based upon the exaggerated emotions.

Intense negative emotion opens the pain gates wide. It decreases the inhibitory signals being produced by the brain and sent from the limbic system down the dorsal horn of the spinal cord. It increases the ratio of excitatory to inhibitory chemicals in the dorsal horn of the spinal cord, which causes pain to increase. You don't just suffer more; you have worse pain. The good news is that this increased pain is completely within your control by using the techniques in this book to tamp down your runaway emotions.

Extreme Negative Emotions Influence Your Pain Behavior

Your emotional response to your pain strongly affects your pain behavior. This tends to be most dramatic when you accentuate your feelings. Letting yourself get caught up in extreme negative emotions exaggerates the severity of the entire pain experience, and makes it more likely that you will exhibit dramatic and even inappropriate pain behaviors. This will damage your credibility with your support system and your doctors. It also wreaks havoc on your ability to function.

By identifying the thoughts that are producing your negative feelings, you can begin to minimize those thoughts and replace them with less distorted ones. You can manage many negative feelings like anger and fear through the relaxation techniques we discussed in Chapter 14.

Many of the strategies that combat negative thoughts also work for negative feelings, since thoughts can produce feelings. The phrase "move your muscles, change your thoughts" is also a strategy for managing strong negative feelings. When you feel miserable and start to dwell on something, try to change positions. Get up, if possible. Move to another location or chair. Try the STAR or STIM techniques. Get involved in a small task or pleasurable activity. Do something that changes your frame of reference so that it breaks the loop that traps you in misery.

Miserable feelings are an inevitable part of the pain experience. However, managing your pain, limitations, and their consequences, also allows you to manage your negative feelings. You can be a scientist and actively work at controlling your feelings rather than just passively responding to them or pushing them away. You will pay the price when you make poor decisions because of your unnecessarily intense emotions. Pain does not make you feel any particular emotion. You can choose how you feel and what you do about it.

Managing my emotions better will help me manage my pain

Insight—I understand that I can actively control my emotions.

Commitment—I am committed to accurately identifying and decreasing negative emotions.

Action—I will be mindful of patterns in my negative emotions and combat the thoughts that cause them.

Now—I think the best change I can make to improve my emotional function is to:

_____

_____

_____

23

When, Why, and How to Take Narcotics

Oral medications are the most common and frequent treatment for chronic pain. For most people in pain, the need for surgeries will end and arise only from new medical problems. Injections will diminish though you may receive an occasional injection for severe pain episodes. Ongoing physical therapy will cease though you may need an occasional course of physical therapy for acute exacerbations of your condition. However, on a long-term basis, the most powerful weapon in the physician's arsenal is oral pain medication.

MATCHING PAIN WITH MEDICATIONS

As much as possible, physicians try to match specific types of medication to specific types of pain. If you have a severe inflammatory process, the best medication is an anti-inflammatory. If you have muscle spasming or tension, a muscle relaxant is best. If you have neuropathic pain, an anticonvulsant may provide pain relief. For migraine headaches, we use triptan medications that minimize the vasoconstriction and brain stem arousal associated with migraine pain. If you have several different types of pain simultaneously, you may require several different types of medications. This treatment approach was defined previously as intellectual polypharmacy.

BASIC FACTS ABOUT NARCOTICS AND CHRONIC PAIN

The grandfather of all pain medications, however, is the narcotic, or opioid. These medications do not address the underlying tissue-based cause of pain, but instead, mask the pain at the level of the brain and the spinal cord. They close pain gates by locking up opioid receptor sites, which inhibits transmission of pain signals to the brain. Whatever doesn't reach the brain isn't pain.

What are Opioids?

The term opioid refers to the original source of opioids, the unripe seedpods of the opium poppy. Medicinal use of opium dates back to ancient Egyptian and Sumerian cultures up to 5,000 years ago. Laudanum is opium dissolved in alcohol and was fashionable in the 1700-1800s. In 1806, the psychoactive and analgesic (pain-relieving) ingredient in opium was isolated and named morphine for Morpheus, the God of Dreams in Greek mythology. Later, another opiate was found in opium, subsequently called codeine.

Heroin, Morphine and Semi-Synthetic Opioids

Heroin is a semi-synthetic variant of morphine developed by the Bayer Company in 1899, a year before they developed aspirin. It has psychoactive and analgesic properties that are two to three times stronger than morphine. Other semi-synthetic opioids are hydromorphone (Dilaudid), Hydrocodone which is synthesized from codeine (Vicodin, Lorcet, Norco), and Oxycodone (Percocet, Roxicodone, OxyContin).

Morphine based analgesics include MS Contin, Kadian, and Avinza. The completely synthetic opioid analgesics include Demerol, Darvon, Fentanyl, Methadone, and Lomotil.

The discovery of the morphine alkaloid in opium in the 1800's eventually led to the discovery of specific receptor sites for opioids. The presence of receptor sites for oral opioids could only be explained if the human body naturally produced opioids as well. The search for naturally occurring opioids led to the discovery of Endorphins. *Endo* stems from the word endogenous or made by the body, *orphin* stems from the word morphine. An endorphin functions like endogenous morphine in that it also blocks pain signals by locking up receptor sites that communicate pain.

The Function of Opioids

Opioids are neither good nor bad in the absolute. Their relative value to a person in pain is determined by a host of factors, including their respective benefits and costs and when, how, and why they are taken. Opioids differ chemically in terms of how they were derived, by the presence of added ingredients, by their molecular composition, and how they are packaged for consumption. These production differences produce functional differences in how quickly opioids enter the blood stream, how well they are absorbed orally, how long they provide pain relief, how much effect they have on central and peripheral nervous system functioning, and how strong or potent they are as analgesics.

Opioids enter the blood stream after administration and the serum level of opioid can be measured. This level indicates the amount of opioid that is available to provide analgesia (pain relief). The higher the opioid serum level, the more analgesia.

The speed with which opioids enter the blood stream and thus provide analgesia is mainly determined by the method of administration. The fastest method of analgesia occurs within a minute. It is achieved by inhaling an opioid into the lungs or the nasal passages. Injection into a vein is the next fastest method followed by sublingual (under the tongue) absorption, both producing analgesia within about three minutes. Oral administration requires twenty to thirty minutes to achieve analgesia while intramuscular or subdermal injection takes thirty to forty minutes. The use of a patch on the skin (transdermally) is the slowest method of analgesia and can require several hours. Interestingly, people with more fatty tissue absorb the opioid faster than those who have low body fat.

Understanding the Duration of Analgesia

Regardless of the administration method, the opioid's chemical composition primarily determines the analgesia duration. Generally, the longer it takes the body to break down an opioid, the longer the duration of analgesia. Comparisons of the length of pain relief for different opioids are usually made based upon the half-life of the opioids, i.e., how long it takes the average body to metabolize half of the active ingredient. Morphine has the shortest half-life of the oral opioids at about two hours. The half-life of hydromorphone (Dilaudid) is two to three hours. Oxycodone (Percocet) and Hydrocodone (Vicodin) have half-lives of about four hours.

The newer continuous-release medications, e.g., MS Contin and OxyContin have half-lives of eight to twelve hours. Methadone has the longest half-life of any of the opioids, up to a full twenty-four hours. This is the main reason why Methadone is effective in helping people to stop using heroin. It minimizes cravings and withdrawal by leveling out the amount of opioid in the blood stream.

Methadone for Long-Term Pain

I'd like to make a quick comment on Methadone. It is a very potent, Schedule 2 opioid with an extremely long half-life. It gets in there and it keeps working, longer than the new, continuous release opioids, such as MS Contin, OxyContin, Kadian, or Avinza. Methadone is also extremely inexpensive because it has been available since 1947—synthesized originally due to a morphine shortage during WWII. It does not provide as much of a peak or mental high as most of the other strong opioids. It has a bad reputation because it has been so heavily associated with heroin withdrawal. However, it is a highly effective opioid, especially for long-term pain. Many of my patients take it with excellent benefit. In my patients, Methadone seems to have a higher side effect potential than some of the other opioids, most commonly from gastrointestinal distress.

THE DIFFERENCE BETWEEN NARCOTIC TOLERANCE AND ADDICTION

The most important fact about all opioids used in pain management is that people develop a tolerance to them and may eventually require higher doses to obtain the same pain relief. Tolerance only develops after opioids have been taken for weeks or months. This does not usually become a problem for people with acute pain but it does for those with chronic pain. Opioids tend to be more effective for acute pain that ends before tolerance develops.

Drug tolerance almost always produces physical withdrawal if the drug is no longer administered. The symptoms of opioid withdrawal can be severe and even life threatening. Symptoms include feeling tense, irritability, nausea, vomiting, headache, sweating, chills, dizziness, weakness, and trembling. The tolerance that patients develop over time and the withdrawal symptoms they experience have led people to describe long-term opioid use as addiction even if the opioid is taken as prescribed. Indeed, most pain programs from the late 1960s until the early 1990s functioned, in part, as detoxification programs in which the first order of business was to withdraw all patients from opioids before the really meaningful work commenced. This strategy was based upon the notion that patients were addicted to their medications, and that they would be better off without them.

However, clinical research through the 1980s created a database suggesting that many patients were able to take opioids long-term and be more functional without the need to escalate their dosage and without their demonstrating any of the symptoms of addiction. In addition, people in pain who took opioids did not seem to experience as much of the recreational effects of opioid use as did their illicit, drug-abusing counterparts. Although these pain patients would show withdrawal symptoms if their opioids were suddenly stopped, and were certainly chemically dependent, they did not abuse the medication or take it for euphoric effect.

In addition, there was no evidence of the physical, psychological, or social impairment necessary for a diagnosis of addiction. In fact, most patients using opioids effectively were found to be more functional and less impaired because of their opioids. These lines of research led to changes in the long-term opioid policy of the American Medical Association and the American Board of Pain Management. Since the mid-1990s, most pain programs have been comfortable prescribing opioids on a long-term basis to selected patients.

SOME PATIENTS SHOULD NOT TAKE NARCOTICS

In the same way that not all patients will benefit from treatment with surgery, injections, or physical therapy, not all patients will benefit from treatment with opioids. A history of chemical dependency or alcoholism makes it far more likely that a patient will abuse opioids and demonstrate formal opioid addiction. A long-term history of depression or anxiety makes it more likely that a patient will use opioids to alleviate their emotional pain.

You are a poor candidate for treatment with opioids if you have been noncompliant with opioids in the past. You should not take opioids if your mental ability is severely impaired by them or if you cannot take them as prescribed. If you have the expectation that opioids should keep you pain free or nearly so, you will not benefit from them. If you have purely neuropathic pain, it is less likely that you will obtain pain relief from opioids. If you develop tolerance quickly and require rapidly escalating doses, you should not take opioids. If you keep running out of your opioids before your refill is due, you should probably be withdrawn from opioids. With all of these problems, it is likely that opioids will not provide you with pain relief in the long run.

Many people assume that opioids have to provide pain relief and that the higher the dose of opioid, the more pain relief they can expect. Some patients assume that if they still have pain, their dose must not be high enough. These patients make a mission out of obtaining the strongest possible opioids in the highest dose they can wrangle. They may be immensely frustrated when they talk to other people who are taking a higher dose than they are prescribed. They assume that they would have more pain relief if they were on the higher dose, too.

If you take opioids for a long time for continuous pain, it is unlikely that your opioid will provide complete pain relief at any point during the day. It is more likely that your opioid will significantly decrease or dull the pain. Patients with the unreasonable expectation of nearly complete pain relief with opioids often become fixated on opioids as the solution to their pain problem. They will invariably assume that their opioid dose is too low because they still have significant pain. Their opioid dosage may consume their thoughts and their discussions with their pain doctors. This will be considered drug seeking, though it is clearly born of a desire for relief from pain. Such patients are not using opioids in a healthy manner.

There are many reasons why a patient may be a poor candidate for ongoing opioid treatment, but the worst candidate for opioids is the person in pain who does not really obtain pain relief and who does not realize it. How is this possible?

SIX REASONS WHY NARCOTICS CAN ACTUALLY INCREASE PAIN

There are six powerful reasons why long-term opioid use may not provide pain relief and can actually increase pain. The first reason is related to opioid tolerance. Figure 15 shows a hypothetical amount of opioid in a person's blood stream that is being taken three times per day with a half-life of three to four hours. When the person in pain first begins taking the opioid, she obtains pain relief at all points along the curve, i.e., with all serum levels of opioid. She receives better pain relief at the higher levels, but she still gets good pain relief at the lower levels.

Figure 15: Variation in Serum Opioid Level Taken Three Times Daily

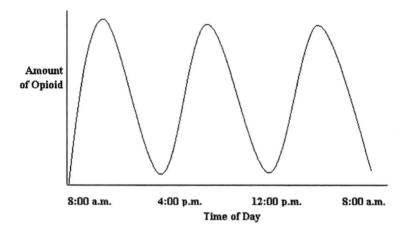

Development of Tolerance to Narcotics

Once the patient in Figure 15 has been on the same dose for a length of time, tolerance develops and she becomes accustomed to the average level of opioid in her blood stream over a twenty-four-hour period. In Figure 16, the average serum level is denoted by the dashed line. At this point, the patient tends to obtain good pain relief only with a serum level that is equal to or greater than she is used to, which is the average amount in her blood stream. Eventually, she is likely to notice that she is obtaining less pain relief from this serum level and the opioid regimen (dosage) that is producing the serum level.

The patient and her doctor need to either accept this decreased pain relief or agree that she will take a higher dose. It is almost inevitable that taking a steady dose of opioid long-term will eventually result in decreased pain relief from that dose. Pain will increase compared to pain immediately following the onset of the dose.

Figure 16: Tolerance and Withdrawal from Daily Opioid Serum Level

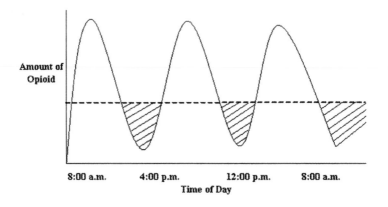

Daily Fluctuations in Narcotic Levels Produce Daily Withdrawal

The second reason why opioids can increase pain is also shown in Figure 16. What do you call the area below the dashed line (average serum level) that is symbolized by the shaded area? This shaded area represents the periods of time when the body has less of the opioid than it is used to or expects. What is it called when you have less of an ingested chemical in your body than you are used to and your body wants more of the chemical to reach equilibrium? It is called withdrawal and you may have experienced this with nicotine, alcohol, or caffeine. If you take short-acting narcotics long enough to develop tolerance, you will experience mild withdrawal as many times in a day as you take the medication. Does this surprise you?

In Figure 16, the patient took the medication three times and was in withdrawal three times, four to eight hours after taking the opioid. Technically, the patient is in withdrawal for nearly as long during the day as she is obtaining good pain relief.

We mentioned some of the symptoms of withdrawal earlier in this chapter and to that list, we can add anxiety and muscle tension—two factors that increase pain in most patients. Increased anxiety and the associated arousal of your nervous system increase neuropathic pain similarly to pouring gasoline on a fire. Increased muscle tension can increase most musculoskeletal pain. Therefore, daily episodes of opioid withdrawal increase chronic pain episodically during each day.

When you have significantly less of almost any drug in your system than you are used to, an additional dose of the drug initially just relieves your withdrawal. It provides little in the way of desired effect, in this case pain relief, until the serum level of the drug begins to approach your average serum level. Then, you begin to obtain the desired effect of good pain relief again.

For a certain period of time each day, withdrawal from opioids may cause you more pain than you would have experienced if you had never begun using opioids at all. Compared to the pain you would have experienced if you never started taking opioids, the peaks of opioid levels may produce less pain (analgesia) while the troughs may produce more pain (withdrawal). With many patients, daily opioid use results in lower pain lows but higher pain highs. You may have greater fluctuations in pain levels because you take opioids.

For example, without opioids, a patient may have an average daily pain level of 60/100 with pain that usually varies between 50 and 70. With opioids, the same patient may still average a 60/100, but with variation between 30 and 90. Unfortunately, many patients in this situation will decide that the solution to their severe pain variability is to increase their dose of narcotic, which may only serve to worsen the variability.

Narcotic Pain Cycles Encourage You to Overdo Physical Exercise

The third reason why opioids can increase chronic pain is that they encourage overdoing, referred to previously as poor pacing and limit setting. Lamar was a patient who had been very active and athletic before his back injury. He was devastated by his injury, pain, and limitations. He was also struck by how much better he felt about himself after he exercised.

On Sunday mornings, he would take a few Vicodin and join his friends on a ten to fifty mile bicycle ride. He felt great, like his old self during his ride and immediately after returning home. Usually by Tuesday afternoon, he could get out of bed again. A few hours of active pleasure notwithstanding, he was in bed or on the couch from Sunday night to Tuesday afternoon with severe pain, during which time dark thoughts filled his head, including anger that his doctor would not increase his opioid dosage.

It may be perfectly reasonable and healthy to use opioids a few times a year to allow yourself to participate in an activity that you would not otherwise be able to join. If family members come into town for an annual visit, or one of your children has a special event, you are welcome to take extra medicine, as long as you are willing to accept the consequences. However, these consequences do not include calling your pain doctor at 3:00 a.m. because you are in severe pain afterward. You caught the bear; you skin it.

The real problem arises when you allow yourself to overdo on a regular basis because you know you will take extra medication after the event. Like Lamar, you may compound matters further by deciding that there is no point in waiting until your pain is severe before taking the extra medicine. If you know you are going to hurt worse, you might be thinking about taking the extra medicine right away to save yourself some pain. What you might have discovered during these activity-induced, severe pain episodes, however, is that oral opioids do not work very well for severe pain episodes.

Figure 17 describes the typical analgesic effects of taking an extra opioid in response to different levels of pain. If you are taking a moderate dose of four opioid tablets per day, then an extra tablet amounts to a 25 percent increase in your total daily dose.

With an excruciating pain level of 100/100 (100 out of 100), an extra tablet may decrease your pain level by 10 to a 90/100, a drop of 10 percent. With a pain level of 90/100, an extra tablet may decrease your pain level by 20 to a 70/100, a drop of 22 percent. With a pain level of 80/100, the extra tablet may decrease your pain level by 30 to a 50/100, a drop of 37 percent. With a pain level of 70/100, the extra tablet may decrease your pain level by 40 to a 30/100, a drop of 57 percent. With a pain level of 60/100, the extra tablet may decrease your pain level by 50 to a 10/100, or a drop of 83 percent.

Figure 17: Opioid Pain Relief

Pain Level Before Opioid	Pain Level After Opioid	Absolute Decrease	Percent of Decrease
100	90	10	10%
90	70	20	22%
80	50	30	37%
70	30	40	57%
60	10	50	83%

The specific numbers above are hypothetical, but reflect reality to make the following point. The less pain you have, the more effective pain medications are, even as a percentage of pain relief. Conversely, the more pain you have, the less pain relief you obtain from an extra dose of opioid, even as a percentage of pain relief.

At pain of 100/100, you get about 10 percent pain relief from an extra opioid tablet. However, the percentage of pain relief increases as pain decreases. At a pain level of 60/100, you get about 83 percent pain relief from an extra opioid tablet. You receive poor pain relief from an extra opioid pill at higher pain levels. This problem is compounded further the higher your dose of daily opioids.

Perhaps you take 100 mgs of OxyContin three times per day, and a 10 mg tab of OxyIR for breakthrough pain three times a day. This is a daily average of 330 mgs. One day you have significantly increased pain of 90/100 after your in-laws visit. You decide to take two extra OxyIRs in addition to your regular single tablet. You have now added 20 mgs of extra Oxycodone, which seems like a lot, except this is an increase of only 6 percent over your daily dose. How much pain relief will you get from an extra 6 percent of opioid for a 90/100 pain level? Very, very little.

Ultimately, the purpose of oral opioids in chronic pain conditions is to improve function and minimize periods of severe pain, not to treat severe pain after it develops. This is more easily done at lower doses of opioids and in the absence of severe overdoing. If you take extra medication on a regular basis because of overdoing, your average daily dose of opioid increases when you account for the extra opioid. You are becoming tolerant to a higher dose, and your regular dose of medication will become less effective in decreasing your baseline pain. This means that you will be stuck with extra pain when you do not take the extra medicine. You will probably be angry and frustrated that your medicine is not working as well as it used to work.

This pattern of taking opioids can lead to what has been described as the narcotic pain cycle. You have pain so you take your opioid. You experience a decrease in your pain that allows you to be more active. You may overdo because you have less pain and you want to maximize accomplishing tasks during the window of pain relief. This creates an even greater increase in pain when the extra opioid wears off. You end up taking more opioids to manage the increased pain. This extra medicine relieves your pain enough that you are again able to increase your activity, perhaps overdoing it again, or perhaps just being able to do the same amount of activity. Over time, this pattern of extra opioid use and overdoing, leads to a higher average amount of medication with the same or increased pain. Again, remember that the higher is your regular dose of opioid, the less effective extra opioids are in managing severe pain.

Relying on Narcotics for Pain Relief Interferes with Using Other Strategies

The fourth reason why opioids can increase pain is an extension of the third reason. If you believe that extra opioids will manage your severe pain, you are less likely to commit to the struggle and effort of learning healthy pacing, limit setting, or other strategies within your Personal Pain Paradigm. Some patients take oral opioids as often as six times per day, on an average of every four hours. That is six decision points per day when you decided to take opioids, and it probably includes several times when you decided to wait.

If you take opioids multiple times a day based upon pain severity, you are spending an enormous amount of your waking day thinking about medication. At the least, it becomes your first "go to" strategy for pain control. Frequently, it becomes your primary strategy for pain control. Why go through the hard work and loss associated with having to learn self-management when it seems like you can just pop a pill?

The bicycle rider, Lamar, inevitably ran out of his medications too soon because he took extra medication most Sundays and Mondays. He was convinced that he was under medicated and that if he were prescribed one more opioid tablet per day, he would be more functional and able to manage his exercise regimen. In truth, an extra pill per day would simply allow him to overdo even more and would probably have increased his average pain.

Using Narcotics Decreases Your Body's Production of Natural Painkillers

The fifth reason why narcotics can eventually increase pain is related to pain tolerance. In the chapter on physical exercise, we commented that how well you tolerate pain is not determined by how much pain you can endure, but by how much pain you actually experience from a given painful stimulus. Numerous factors affect pain tolerance but chief among them is how many endogenous opiates (endorphins and enkephalins) your body can produce and send to opiate receptors. The more of these naturally produced painkillers your body makes, the less pain you will have. We noted further that aerobic exercise is the best way to encourage the body to produce natural opiates. Unfortunately, taking synthetic opioid medications on a regular basis discourages the body from producing endorphins and enkephalins, based in part on the principle of homeostasis.

Homeostasis is the life organizing principle that living tissue needs to keep an internal steady state or equilibrium to sustain life. In humans, too much potassium or too little water can affect homeostasis enough to cause death. A secondary tenet of homeostasis is that chemicals that the body takes in regularly from the environment can become integrated into the homeostatic balance, i.e., the body becomes accustomed to consuming them. Symptoms of withdrawal will result if the chemical is unavailable. A third tenet is that if your body stops using something internally, it will stop producing it or the associated physical structure will waste away.

For instance, if you do not use the muscles in your low back and legs because you are on the couch 24/7, your back and leg muscles will weaken and atrophy. If you eat red meat very infrequently, your body becomes less effective at digesting it, and you may experience stomach upset when you do eat red meat.

Remember that the natural opiates your body manufactures and the synthetic opiates you are prescribed from your doctor are very similar. They travel to the same receptor sites and work in the same way to activate the receptors and decrease pain. Using the lock-and-key model, the two types of opiates are keys that compete for the same keyholes to lock the doors to pain. And the opiates you take orally overwhelm the endogenous ones your body makes—they almost always win the competition.

You may know that, in the reproductive process, thousands of sperm compete to be the one that fertilizes the single egg. We know what happens to the winner; it becomes your child. What happens to the losers? They are unceremoniously flushed out of your system. The same thing happens to endogenous opiates when they lose the lock-and-key competition to oral opiates. They are flushed out. Consistent with the principles of homeostasis, because your body is not using its own opiates much, over time it decreases or nearly ceases production of them. Decreased amounts of endorphins and enkephalins literally and biochemically decrease your pain tolerance since you will experience more pain from a given painful stimulus.

Chronic opioid use inevitably decreases pain tolerance by decreasing production of natural opiates. If chronic opioid use is combined with a lack of physical exercise, there is nothing encouraging your body to produce endorphins and enkephalins, except the pain itself. The lengthy use of even moderate doses of opioids, combined with minimal exercise, can result in ever more severe decreases in biochemical pain tolerance. This is often a major contributor to the development of disabling, total body pain stemming from a specific injury.

Chronic opioid use inevitably decreases pain tolerance. In the absence of regular exercise, your decreased pain tolerance will result in increased pain for which you may want to take more opioids. This chain of events is a disaster.

Now we can revisit the goals of pain management and make some additional statements. We noted that the goal of pain treatment and management was to decrease pain, increase activity, or both. Perhaps the most important goal of chronic opioid use is to increase physical exercise without overdoing. At least initially, using opioids to promote exercise is much more helpful to self-management than to promote general activity throughout the day. If you have chronic pain and take opioids, it is imperative that daily physical exercise gets the best part of your day.

A common question at this point in pain class is, "If I stop taking opioids, will my body resume producing higher levels of endorphins and enkephalins?" The answer is yes, but it can take three to six months to normalize, which is a period that can be shortened if you begin exercising. In the intervening time, you would need to aggressively persevere with non-medical strategies for self-management of pain.

Narcotics Can Increase Chronic Pain Suffering

The sixth reason why chronic opioid use can increase pain is related to the suffering aspect of the pain experience. Sometimes I summarize this in pain class by saying with a smile "Opioids can make you stupid." They can and do affect attention, concentration, short-term memory, perseverance, organization, and the infamous ability to operate heavy machinery. They can blunt or dull your emotional experience and thereby increase your depression. They can suck the energy and motivation right out of you and compel you to become a couch potato. Furthermore, they can produce a myriad of unpleasant physical side effects.

Daily high doses of opioids can grossly compromise your doctor's ability to manage painful procedures. Let's be honest. If you take 400 mgs of OxyContin or MS Contin daily and you undergo a spinal fusion surgery, your doctors will simply not be able to keep you comfortable for the first several weeks post surgically. You might need 800 to 2400 mgs of opioid for a month or two following surgery to effectively manage this acute, post surgical pain. Since this dose of opioids could be fatal or end your doctor's career, you simply will not be prescribed such a high dose.

Regarding the caution about operating heavy machinery while taking opioids, many people take that to mean that they cannot legally drive a motor vehicle. The law states that you are allowed to take any dose of legal opioid as prescribed and drive a motor vehicle. However, you are not allowed to be intoxicated or obviously impaired due to your opioid use. With alcohol, impaired is defined in The United States as a blood alcohol level of about .08 to .1, even though some individuals might be trashed at .06, and others might not be affected much at .15. There is no comparable scale for opioids. This makes decisions regarding your being "under the influence" up to the assessment of law enforcement officers and a judge, subsequently. If you take a prescribed dose, the burden of proof is on the law enforcement officer or judge to document that you were impaired.

You need to assess your driving safety. Generally, people who have just begun taking opioids will demonstrate some decreased cognitive and motor skill function until and unless they develop a tolerance to the medication. On the other hand, people who have severe pain demonstrate significant impairment on those same measures related to driving performance. Some studies have suggested that moderate doses of opioids for chronic pain that are tolerated well actually improve cognitive and motoric function as they decrease pain.

Decisions about receiving chronic opioid therapy are complicated and should be based on assessment of all the relative benefits and costs of opioid treatment. If you are certain that you are too impaired to drive on your opioid regimen, this means one of four things. You may not have developed tolerance yet and may need to give your body more time. You may be far less impaired on a different opioid and need to switch medications. You may be taking too high a dose and need to decrease it. Or, you may react in an unusual way to opioids that prevents you from ever driving safely while taking any type of opioid at any dose. In this last case, you should not take opioids, since you are less functional while taking them.

Due to the potential complications with chronic opioid use, a patient's self-report of pain relief is not the best measure of opioid effectiveness. We have discussed how a patient may receive tremendous pain relief two hours after taking an opioid and actually end up with more chronic pain and decreased activity because of his opioid regimen. Thus, the best measure of the effectiveness of opioids is the presence of increased physical, social, pleasurable, and productive activity.

Research literature strongly encourages physicians to use changes in activity and functioning as the primary index of opioid effectiveness. The people in your support system may be able to provide you with healthy, constructive feedback about whether you seem more or less functional taking them.

How Taking Narcotics Effectively Can Decrease Chronic Pain

In spite of the fact that there are six major reasons that opioids may not decrease pain and can actually increase pain, many people take opioids with good benefit in terms of pain and increased daily activity. There are several strategies for minimizing the potential negative effects of opioids and maximizing their benefit. If you are able to take opioids only a few times a week or less and practice good self-management, you will avoid all of the potential problems with opioids. You can take them as you choose.

Most people who take opioids for at least moderate chronic pain take them daily. With the vast majority of people, opioids should be taken on a time-contingent basis and not a pain-contingent basis. This means taking your regular opioids at the same time every day regardless of pain level.

Many patients pride themselves on only taking their opioids when the pain is so terrible they cannot stand it anymore. However, we know that opioids are less effective with severe pain. A better goal is to use opioids in concert with self-management to try to prevent severe pain. If you take opioids every day, or almost daily, it is far better to take them on a schedule rather than just as needed. Scheduled doses will level out the concentration of opioid in your blood stream. This means that the variation in your blood serum level is minimized, i.e., you have smaller peaks and valleys. Time contingent dosing takes the time-consuming decision-making out of the process. It also prevents you from using opioids to overdo and precludes a potential narcotic pain cycle. It gives your body the best opportunity to eliminate unhealthy mental and emotional responses to opioids.

How often you take a daily opioid should be determined by your unique needs and lifestyle while considering the half-life of your medication. Research has consistently demonstrated that with daily opioid use, pain relief improves the steadier you maintain your opioid serum level.

Figure 18 shows the theoretically perfect serum level for chronic opioids as a horizontal line. This steady serum level provides the maximal amount of pain relief and increased function from a given type and dose of opioid. A flat serum level means that you are continually receiving the average amount of opioid to which your body has become accustomed. You obtain pain relief throughout the day.

Without the valleys in opioid serum level, you avoid the usual daily episodes of withdrawal symptoms caused by having less opioid in your system than your body expects. Without the peaks in opioid serum level, you avoid the sudden, brief decreases in pain that promote severe overdoing, i.e., extremely poor limit setting.

Figure 18: Ideal Daily Opioid Serum Level

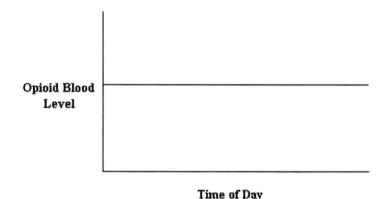

For medications with a short half-life, like Vicodin, you would benefit from taking the medication about every four hours to level out the serum concentration in your blood stream. For the continuous release medicines like MS Contin or OxyContin, a dose of two to three times per day provides fairly steady serum levels. The Duragesic patch (Fentanyl) tends to produce the steadiest opioid serum level of any of the self-administered opioids in large measure due to the transdermal route of administration.

If you take opioids several times per day, level dosing provides maximal pain relief. The severe fluctuations in opioid serum levels inevitably cause problems. However, there is a powerful reason why you may resist this type of dosing in the belief that it does not provide the best pain relief.

How do you know if your pain medication is working? The simplest and most common way to assess pain relief from oral opioids is to determine if you experience a dramatic decrease in pain soon after taking the medication. Most of us have been using this method of evaluating analgesia for decades, whether the medication is aspirin for a headache or morphine for kidney stones. We evaluate how much pain relief we get and how quickly we get it after taking a medication.

Unfortunately, rapid, dramatic pain relief after taking an opioid occurs only when there is a huge spike or peak in the opioid serum level. But, with level dosing, you never get this spike. You do not get the dramatic, "Ahhhh! That feels better!" This is why many patients are convinced that Vicodin helps their pain more than MS Contin. The serum level with Vicodin peaks quickly and since it has a relatively short half-life, patients are probably in withdrawal whenever they take another dose. Compared to continuous-release opioids, the rapid-release opioids produce greater peaks and valleys with the same frequency of dosing.

For many patients, a compromise opioid regimen calls for taking a continuous-release medication two to three times per day with the option of taking a rapid-release medication a few times per day as needed for breakthrough pain. The rapid-release medication is usually taken at a much lower dose than the continuous-release, so it provides a little pain relief without causing the problematic spikes in serum opioid levels. As a rule, you should only take breakthrough medicine as often as you take your continuous-release opioid. If you find that you must take your breakthrough medicine more frequently, your doctor probably needs to increase your dose of continuous-release medication.

STRATEGIES FOR OPIOID CESSATION

After you have been taking opioids for an extended period of time, you and your doctor may decide that you should stop taking them. Perhaps they provide inadequate pain relief to compensate for the side effects. Maybe you are incapable of taking them as prescribed and frequently run out of your opioid long before the next refill. Perhaps your pain has been significantly reduced through other methods and you no longer need to take opioids.

Regardless of the reason for opioid cessation, many patients report that they have much less pain after terminating opioid use. This should not be surprising given the six problems with opioids we discussed previously. Yet, I am sometimes surprised when I see a patient a month after he has stopped an opioid regimen. The patient may look like a different person—smiling, more alert, and apparently suffering less in every way. The transformation can be remarkable.

There are several strategies for opioid cessation. The first is gradual tapering over many weeks or months to minimize any withdrawal symptoms. This requires that the patient be able to stick to a lengthy tapering regimen. The benefit is that the process is conducted on an outpatient basis with minimal expense.

The second strategy is to detoxify the patient over a week or less. Many hospitals provide this service on an inpatient basis, often using the mask and fade technique. The opioid is given in liquid form in decreasing amounts using the same amount of liquid so the patient has no idea how much opioid he is receiving. Non-narcotic medications are used liberally to ease symptoms of withdrawal. These often include benzodiazepines, such as Valium, and anti-nausea drugs like Compazine.

A relatively new type of opioid cessation program is called Accelerated Neuro-regulation, or Rapid Detox. My colleague, Clifford Bernstein, M.D., is the Medical Director of the Waissman Institute, a hospital-based program in Los Angeles, California. He stated, "We can accelerate the detox process over a twelve-hour period while patients are in an induced sleep and provide antagonist medications to eliminate withdrawal symptoms. Our success rate is much higher than with traditional medical detox."

Very recently, two new drugs were FDA approved in the United States for use with opioid dependency and detoxification on an in-office basis. Subutex is buprenorphine hydrochloride, a weak opioid or partial opioid agonist, which reduces withdrawal symptoms and blocks the effects of subsequently administered opiates. Suboxone is a combination of buprenorphine and naloxone, the latter an opioid antagonist that reverses the effects of opioids. These medications minimize withdrawal symptoms and maximize compliance with detox as they interfere with the effects of any other opioids a patient might take. There is no point in taking opioids if they are rendered ineffective.

If you are considering opioid cessation, you should talk to your physician about the various options. Your doctor may not be aware of some of the newer programs. For information about any of the programs discussed above, you can access our web site at www.MyPainReliefDoc.com or contact me at PACE, Inc., P.O. Box 6599, Irvine, CA 92616.

After this chapter, I hope you are in a better position to evaluate the appropriateness of your opioid regimen and can assess the relative advantages and disadvantages. You cannot simply focus on your awareness of decreased pain after taking the pill. Are you more active and functional now than before taking opioids? When your opioids change, are you more or less functional on the new medication? With level dosing, you may have better insight into pain relief by keeping a pain and activity record in your TAAP journal before, during, and after the initiation of, or change in, an opioid regimen. If your doctor does not prescribe the stronger or continuous-release opioids, you may wish to request a referral to a doctor who does.

Do not hesitate to ask the people around you what they have noticed in terms of your apparent pain, function, and side effects. Many hundreds of thousands of people around the world use prescription opioids very effectively to improve their activity and function and to decrease pain. Conversely, many tens of thousands of people around the world would have less pain and suffering if they stopped using prescription opioids. The decisions you make about opioids may be the most important for your long-term medical care. Be fully informed and choose wisely.

I will decide scientifically if, when, why, and how I will take opioids

Insight—I realize now that opioids can either decrease or increase my pain.

Commitment—I am committed to using opioids effectively or not at all.

Action—If I choose to take opioids daily, I will take them on a time-contingent basis, keeping my blood levels as steady as possible.

Now—I will stop using as my main assessment of pain relief how much better I feel thirty minutes to two hours after I take my opioid.

24

How Your Lifestyle Can Affect Your Pain

An unhealthy lifestyle can worsen your pain and sabotage your rehabilitation. Your medical providers will probably not involve themselves significantly in most lifestyle changes. However, your habits regarding non-prescription chemicals, sleep, and nutrition are largely within your control.

CHEMICAL DEPENDENCY AND SUBSTANCE USE WITH CHRONIC PAIN

Obviously, it is a bad idea to use non-prescription drugs like cocaine, PCP, methamphetamine, ecstasy, or LSD, etc. It is bad for your general health and interferes with your brain's ability to cope with pain and your body's ability to improve function and activity. If you use these drugs sporadically, just know that you are playing with fire and will burn if you continue. If you use these drugs regularly, you will never be able to gain control over pain until you stop. Talk to your doctor. Consider a substance abuse program. Attend some type of narcotics anonymous program.

Alcohol Use with Chronic Pain

Alcohol use is more complicated. It is not healthy to consume more than two to three ounces of alcohol daily, about the amount of alcohol in two shots of liquor, two glasses of wine, or two beers. There is some evidence to suggest that drinking a glass or two of red wine daily may be healthy. If you drink more than this amount daily, it is probably impairing your mental function, energy, mood, relationships, and ability to manage pain. If you describe your drinking as less than it is to your doctors, or have been in trouble for drinking in the past year or two, you probably have an alcohol problem.

Alcohol is one of the oldest analgesics in the world. The truth is that if you drink enough, it will help with your pain. It may kill you, or make you wish you were dead the next day, but in large doses, alcohol is an effective painkiller. Even infrequent use of alcohol in amounts large enough to bring significant pain relief will negatively affect your health. However, if you are not taking any medications and do not have a history of alcohol or chemical dependency, an ounce or two of alcohol at the end of a day is not terribly unhealthy regardless of your pain status.

On the other hand, if you are taking muscle relaxants, opioids, benzodiazepines, sleeping medication, or anti-anxiety medication, drinking alcohol will have a synergistic effect and make you much more groggy, lethargic, and otherwise impaired (or dead) beyond what would be expected for either alcohol or medications alone. Candidly, it also brings better pain relief than either does alone. If you have tried combining alcohol and pain medicine, you know this. However, the safety and consistency of interactions between alcohol and pain medicine is poor. Alcohol interferes with the function of antidepressants and antibiotics as well as other medications. If you are taking almost any medication for your pain problem or related sequelae, you are better off minimizing your consumption of alcohol.

Marijuana Use with Chronic Pain

Marijuana is another analgesic that has been around for many centuries. Cannabis is currently and rather recently illegal in many countries including the United States. Still, probably about 10-20 percent of my patients admit to trying marijuana as a pain reliever for their chronic pain. Most of them report significant pain relief. Some comment that it is their most effective pain reliever.

I take the position that marijuana is neither intrinsically good nor bad. Like all pain relievers, the usefulness of "pot" as an analgesic depends on the relative benefits and costs. A practical disadvantage in many countries is that it is illegal and a user can be sent to prison. Regular use of marijuana is documented to impair attention, concentration, short-term memory, and initiative. After administration, marijuana remains in your system much longer than opioids. The vast majority of pain doctors will not prescribe it because they rightly fear harming their reputations or ending their careers.

Although marijuana is available in tablet form as Marinol, the vast majority of patients who have compared the analgesic effects of smoking marijuana with swallowing Marinol tablets report that smoking is many times more effective for pain relief. Though marijuana does not contain nicotine, it does contain many of the same cancer-causing ingredients found in tobacco, and we assume, similar health risks if smoked.

The United States federal government opines that there are no proven medical benefits for smoking marijuana, thus justifying its categorization as a Schedule 1 drug. In the current political "war on drugs" climate, the government is also not authorizing any clinical research to assess the analgesic effects of smoking marijuana. As long as the federal bureaucrats and politicians make research on marijuana smoking illegal, they can claim there are no proven medical benefits and smoking marijuana will remain both illegal and nonprescription—a Catch 22 of potentially monumental and tragic proportions. They choose politics over science and reason. You make your own choice.

Nicotine Use with Chronic Pain

Most relevant to chronic pain are the legal stimulant chemicals, especially nicotine and caffeine. Obviously, cigarette smoking carries hundreds of health risks unrelated to pain. However, nicotine has two other characteristics that increase pain and compromise rehabilitation. First, nicotine impairs the body's ability to transport oxygen, including to the bones, muscles, and even the brain itself. This can be such a severe problem that many spine surgeons will not perform spinal-fusion surgery on actively smoking patients because of the unacceptably high failure rate. The spine never fuses properly because the fusion material and vertebra do not receive enough oxygenated blood to create fusion.

By impairing oxygen transport, nicotine also impairs the body's ability to rehabilitate. It makes muscles weaker and the body more easily fatigued. If you are trying to exercise and increase strength, endurance, and range of motion, nicotine is the greatest chemical barrier to those healthy changes. Again, the relevant body parts do not receive enough oxygen to grow, heal, or become stronger.

Second, nicotine is an extremely powerful stimulant and smoking is the most potent method of administering any chemical. When a smoker inhales smoke, the heart rate increases within a few seconds, reflecting increased arousal of the autonomic nervous system. Increased muscle tension is one symptom of increased arousal, which almost inevitably increases most chronic pain conditions. Even if your pain is purely neuropathic, the increased autonomic arousal caused by nicotine will increase your neuropathic pain.

Caffeine Consumption with Chronic Pain

Few stimulant chemicals have the oxygen sapping properties of nicotine, but most stimulants, including caffeine, can eventually make you more fatigued. You know that you feel more awake after you take a stimulant, hence, drinking coffee in the morning. But when the stimulation wears off, you become more fatigued than you would have been if you had never taken the stimulant. This is a rebound effect.

Many people who drink a lot of coffee in the morning notice a late morning or early afternoon crash when they feel tired. Caffeine is a powerful stimulant and the amount of caffeine in coffee is high. If you have more than a single cup of coffee, or caffeinated tea, it is almost inevitable that you will experience some rebound-induced lethargy during the day. You may counteract this by consuming more caffeine, perhaps through soda. At this point, you are officially chemically dependent, driven to continue consuming caffeine to maintain your function and avoid withdrawal and fatigue.

Most people are not familiar with all the products other than coffee that contain caffeine. Black teas have caffeine, as does chocolate or cocoa of any kind. There is caffeine in many pain relievers including Midol, Anacin, Excedrin, etc. Many migraine medications contain caffeine. All regular colas and some non-cola sodas contain caffeine. You should assess how much caffeine you consume in any form on a daily basis.

HOW TO IMPROVE SLEEP AND DECREASE CHRONIC PAIN

Sleep disturbance is the rule not the exception for people in pain. It is difficult to fall asleep when you hurt because you may not be able to find a genuinely comfortable position. It can be almost impossible to stay asleep, because remaining in any one position for six to eight hours, even lying down, is likely to escalate pain and awaken you. You may have other problems that awaken you during the night, like the urge to urinate, and your pain makes it more difficult to fall back asleep each time.

We know that chronic pain can produce both anxiety and depression. Anxiety is mostly associated with difficulty falling asleep while depression is mostly associated with early morning awakening. Further, sleep is compromised by the inactivity and lack of exercise common to people in pain.

The quality of your sleep is just as important as your amount of sleep. You can get eight to ten hours of sleep and still be exhausted if it was of poor quality. There are four stages of sleep, handily named Stages 1-4. The first stage is falling asleep where you are awake but drifting comfortably. The second stage is light sleep during which you are easily aroused. Stages 3 and 4 are considered deep sleep.

It takes about ninety minutes to cycle through all four stages, which means you cycle through the stages about four to six times in an eight-hour sleep period. However, after the first cycle, you do not return to Stage 1 as it is replaced by a different stage referred to as REM sleep for the rapid eye movements that are frequent during this stage. About 95 percent of people report dreaming when they are wakened during the REM stage while their eyes are moving. In Stage 2, during each cycle, you are aroused relatively easily by pain, bathroom urges, noise, etc. When you awaken during the night, it is most often during Stage 2 sleep.

If you awaken once or twice during the night, and fall asleep again immediately, your sleep quality is not affected much. However, if you wake up multiple times during the night, seemingly tossing and turning all night, you may not be getting enough REM or deep sleep. Adequate REM and deep sleep are necessary to feel rested and to function well during the day. Some people who are experimentally or otherwise deprived of deep sleep, develop symptoms very similar to Fibromyalgia (FMS), leading some researchers to believe FMS is related to or caused by a sleep disorder. This could explain why FMS often develops after a physical injury and subsequent pain, the latter usually producing sleep disturbance.

There are many nutritional supplements using herbs and medication precursors that encourage restful sleep. Tryptophan is the chemical in turkey that makes you sleepy after consuming mass quantities. This chemical is converted into 5-hydroxytryptophan (5-HTP) and then into Serotonin, the nonspecific neurotransmitter that improves mood, pain, and sleep. Many effective sleep aids contain either Tryptophan or 5-HTP. Other herbal sleep aids promote sleep and drowsiness by autonomic quieting and muscular relaxation.

Satiete is among the best natural sleep aids containing 5-HTP. An excellent calming and relaxing sleep aid is Sleep-Tite which contains valerian, kava kava, skullcap, and chamomile to encourage restful sleep. These and various other supplements can be ordered online at www.MyPainReliefDoc.com.

Your doctor can and should attend to your sleep problem. This is one of the most important functions of a pain doctor. On a short-term or occasional basis, your doctor can prescribe formal sleeping medicine, e.g., Halcion (Triazolam),

Restoril (Temazepam), Ambien (Zolpidem), Xyrem (Sodium Oxybate), or Sonata (Zaleplon). However, these medicines are generally not meant for daily or long-term use. Your body habituates to them, since they are sedating-anxiolytic type medications, and you develop a tolerance to them. Also, your sleep becomes even more impaired after a long period of use when you do not take them.

If you need sleeping medicine daily, you are probably better off with a low dose, sedating antidepressant, e.g., Amitriptyline or Nortriptyline. These medications are more likely to help with nightly sleep disturbance on a long-term basis than the anxiolytic type. If you are taking opioids or muscle relaxants, you may request a dose of either medication at bedtime to improve your sleep further. The less medication you take during the day, the more benefit you will receive from a sleep medication. If you take opioids, muscle relaxants, anti-convulsants, antidepressants, and anxiolytic medications in large doses during the day, a mild sleeping medication may be like "spitting in the ocean"—it simply will not be noticed.

What you do to help yourself sleep is probably more important than your doctor's help. Daily exercise at the comfortable limits of your tolerance is most important and more valuable than being active throughout the day. As much as possible, your exercise should be scheduled when you tend to be at your best physically and psychologically. For most people, this occurs early in the day. Structure your activities so that you arise and go to bed at the same time each day. Avoid long naps.

If you are exhausted during the day, you can take a short, thirty to forty-five minute nap, but not much later than about 1:00 p.m. Let yourself wind down for about an hour before bedtime, minimizing stimulation, noise, and work. Avoid taking any stimulants after 6:00 p.m. including chocolate. Let your bed be a strong cue for sleep. Refrain from reading, eating, or watching television in bed. Your bed is for sleeping and sexual activity, period—not at the same time, of course.

If you do not fall asleep after about twenty minutes, get out of bed, and do something non-stimulating, such as a relaxation exercise or some light reading. This is not the time to plan the next day. If you awaken at night, give yourself twenty minutes to fall asleep again, then get out of bed, do something non-stimulating, and try to sleep again. Do not use alcohol habitually to help yourself sleep because it can impair the quality of your sleep.

THE IMPORTANCE OF GOOD NUTRITION WITH CHRONIC PAIN

Weight management and nutrition are complementary in promoting pain management. Weight gain places additional stress on already sore muscles, ligaments, and joints. If you have pain in your spine, knees, or hips, gaining weight in your stomach or chest strains your body even more. If you have gained more than 20 percent of your body weight and your pain is musculoskeletal, you can be almost assured that losing weight will decrease your pain. Good nutrition is an important strategy in maintaining a healthy weight, but it has other, pain-related benefits as well.

It has been said, "Garbage in, garbage out." This describes nutrition perfectly, since food is the fuel for everything we do. Avoid radical and fad diets. Your eating habits should be healthy and sustainable over the course of your life. You do not need to lose the weight in four weeks that you gained over months or years. Remember that you are working on a hundred other things, too.

You should eat at least two servings a day from the five basic food groups: fruits, vegetables, grains and pasta, dairy, and lean meats, with about 70-80 percent of calories from protein and complex carbohydrates and about 30 percent from fat. Lean red meat is perfectly healthy in moderation. Fresh foods are healthier than processed foods. Extremely low carbohydrate diets can promote weight loss but may not be as healthy over a lifetime as a more balanced approach to eating.

Protein is the building block of physical rehabilitation and increasing strength. You must consume enough protein, a minimum of three servings a day. This gives your body the fuel it needs to become stronger.

Water is the single most important molecule in the cells of your body. Performance decreases significantly with even a small percentage change in cellular water content. It is extremely important that you keep yourself adequately hydrated, which means a minimum of three twelve-ounce glasses of water per day.

As a rule, avoid refined sugar. You do not have to be a monk, but make sweets a treat, not a daily habit. Sugar causes swings in blood glucose levels. At the low end of the pendulum, you will have low energy and maybe even negative moods that can severely affect your pain, exercise, and activity level. Being moderate with salt, sodium, saturated fats, and cholesterol improves health, performance, and longevity. Fruits are high in sugar content, and you probably should not eat more than two servings daily.

Over the course of a lifetime, it is extremely difficult to obtain maximally healthy or even adequate nutrition from food alone. This recognition has lead to an explosion in research and development of natural food supplements. There are many hundreds of companies selling thousands of products in this unregulated market. The best supplements are listed in the Physician's Desk Reference for Nonprescription Drugs and Dietary Supplements. You are safest with companies that have been in business for at least a decade with FDA approved manufacturing facilities. There are dozens of companies that provide high quality supplements directed toward specific health concerns. Many of the supplements I recommend to my patients are manufactured by Wellness International (WIN), an established company with a solid product line. You can review a list of nutritional supplements and order WIN supplements at www.MyPainReliefDoc.com.

Numerous research studies have suggested that all adults should take a daily multivitamin and mineral supplement. These supplements allow your body to function at its best and to extract the best nutrients from the food you eat. Chronic pain severely stresses the body and challenges most of the organ systems, especially musculoskeletal, cardiovascular, gastrointestinal, and immune. Phyto-Vite from Wellness International is an excellent multi-vitamin and multi-mineral with strong antioxidant properties formulated to enhance prolonged absorption of nutrients.

Remember, protein is the building block of physical rehabilitation and recovery. It has been estimated that over half the world's population does not consume enough protein, even in cultures with adequate financial resources. The process of managing chronic pain requires even greater protein intake since building strength in bones and muscles requires extra protein. There are hundreds of protein-based supplements including those made by EAS, Optimum Nutrition, and Met-Rx. I use and recommend Pro-Extreme by Wellness International, to be taken once per day, often as a meal replacement, to ensure adequate protein levels throughout the day.

Weight Management with Chronic Pain

Most people in pain gain weight following pain onset because of decreased activity and exercise, and poor eating habits. Weight is determined primarily by your metabolic rate and caloric intake. Your metabolic rate is the rate at which you burn calories at rest. The higher your metabolic rate, the less you will weigh with a given caloric intake and the more calories you can consume to maintain a given weight. The goal of any weight loss program is to increase metabolic rate and decrease caloric intake.

Your metabolic rate is increased when you exercise and when you eat because it takes energy to exercise and digest food. The more often you eat, the more your metabolic rate increases. By eating only once or twice a day, your digestive system is relatively inactive most of the day. This digestive inactivity slows your metabolism. If you eat multiple times a day, you are constantly burning calories to digest food, thereby raising your metabolism. Of course, the only way you can eat frequently and not increase calories is to eat small meals. Healthy eating means eating five to six times a day, about every three waking hours, described as three to four small meals and two healthy snacks.

Some people eat when they are bored, stressed, miserable, lonely, or depressed. These are common symptoms of people in pain. Practice other healthy eating strategies. Try to resist unhealthy foods in the grocery store. When it is time to eat, do it at the kitchen table, not in the bedroom, living room, family room, or den. Eat slowly and give yourself time to feel full. Serve small portions and keep serving dishes off the table. The more water you drink throughout the day, the less food you will want to eat.

Nutritional supplements can strongly support weight management and weight loss. These supplements are generally based upon one of four major strategies for weight loss:

- Increasing metabolic rate

- Decreasing calories with meal replacements

- Suppressing appetite

- Blocking absorption of fats or carbohydrates.

Stimulant-type chemicals will increase metabolism and include ephedra or caffeine type stimulants or other thermogenic chemicals such as creatine, chromium picolinate, chromium polynicotinate, and Pyruvate. Nutritional drinks like SlimFast and Ensure were designed to be meal replacements. Appetite suppressant supplements include the newest, Hoodia Gordonii, an extract from the South African plant. Fat blockers include Chitosan and Xenical (Orlistat).

The Biolean line of weight loss supplements from Wellness International, used in conjunction with their Pro-Extreme and Satiete products, compels weight loss through all four approaches to weight loss. Ultimately, this is the most powerful nonprescription strategy for weight loss. You can browse some of your neighborhood health and nutrition stores or review and order over the Internet. Further information about supplements that are specific to your health needs is available at www.MyPainReliefdoc.com.

CONSTIPATION WITH CHRONIC PAIN

Constipation is not often discussed but is a common health problem for people in pain. Lack of exercise, inactivity, infrequent eating, and medications can all contribute to infrequent bowel movements. Use of opioids severely worsens this problem. Healthy people move their bowels daily. However, it is not unusual for people in pain to average only two to three bowel movements per week. Many people in pain have gone a week or longer without a bowel movement. Due to poor regularity, fecal matter can build up in the colon, causing toxic effects, which have been known to produce symptoms of bloating, pain, or flu-like sensations.

The most important strategies for easing constipation are to increase activity, exercise, frequency of eating, and water consumption. Minimizing the use of opioids and other CNS depressing medications will also help. Anything that speeds up metabolic activity will increase bowel movement frequency.

There are various nonprescription supplements for alleviating constipation. They are categorized based upon the mechanism of action. Bulk-forming laxatives soften and increase the volume of your stools, e.g., Fibercon, Benefiber, and Citrucel. Stimulant laxatives increase the rate of digestion and elimination, e.g., Dulcolax. Osmotic laxatives increase the amount of water in your stools making them softer and easier to pass, e.g., Milk of Magnesia. Many over-the-counter laxatives are not therapeutic with chronic constipation and can result in dependence upon the medication. Supplements that are more sophisticated can aid digestion as well as soften and increase stool bulk, e.g., STEPHAN Relief through Wellness International.

Your doctor can prescribe medications for constipation including Senokot or Miralax. More severe constipation that lasts many days may require suppository treatments or drinking a liquid medication designed to cleanse the colon, e.g, GoLytely, a misnomer if ever there was one.

Constipation is a serious health problem that can be life threatening and even require surgery. If you go longer than five or six days without a bowel movement, you should contact your doctor immediately. Moving your bowels is a completely normal function that you can be comfortable discussing with your doctor.

SEX AND CHRONIC PAIN

Sexual activity is almost inevitably affected by chronic pain. For most people in pain, many sexual activities make pain worse—not a great inducement to be sexual. Your partner may become afraid of hurting you when you are sexual. Injury to some of the nerves in the low back can inhibit erection. Your sex drive can be profoundly diminished by medications, pain, depression, anxiety, anger, inactivity, and decrements in testosterone. Arousal for both men and women can be affected as well, leading to problems with lubrication or sustaining an erection. Finally, orgasm can be made difficult to achieve or much less intense.

Sexual dissatisfaction is one of the major contributors to marital conflict in families with chronic pain. You and your partner may need to be creative and willing to try new things that make sex easier, less painful, or simply more fun. For many heterosexual couples, this may mean de-emphasizing intercourse and experimenting with other types of lovemaking. Open, honest discussion is essential.

There are significant physical health benefits associated with sexual activity beyond a sense of wellness or intimacy. If you have difficulty in any area of sexual health, you should discuss this with your doctor. There are medications, techniques, and even surgeries that can be beneficial. Many pain physicians can help you understand how to manage these problems, though you may ultimately benefit from a consultation with a gynecologist, urologist, or psychologist for more advanced care.

MAINTAINING A HEALTHY LIFESTYLE

A healthy lifestyle is important for everyone. This includes control over chemicals, sleep, weight, and nutrition. For people who are pain free, an unhealthy lifestyle may effect long-term health mainly and cause only minor inconvenience on a daily basis. For people in pain, however, an unhealthy lifestyle can have a powerful effect on daily pain and function. There are so many aspects of your pain, over which you have no control, that it can be very comforting, indeed, to know that you can control your lifestyle, and thereby reduce your pain and suffering. Over the next twenty-four hours, monitor your lifestyle habits and document them in your TAAP journal.

My pain is affected by my lifestyle more than I realized

Insight—I understand that stimulants, alcohol, obesity, and poor sleep can increase my pain.

Commitment—I am committed to maintaining a healthier lifestyle including taking a multivitamin.

Action—I will change my intake of unhealthy items and practice a healthy sleep pattern, good nutrition, and a supplement regimen.

Now—I think it would be healthy for me to take the following types of supplements:_____

_____

_____.

25

Identifying Motivational Challenges to Rehabilitation

With chronic pain, your motivation to rehabilitate yourself is not as straight forward as you might think. You need to distinguish between your motivation to recover completely and your motivation to recover as much as possible. In particular, your motivation to minimize your own suffering can be complicated.

I have never met a person in pain who did not want to be pain free, who would not have traded their current life in pain for the quality of life they had before their pain began. However, with chronic pain, complete and total recovery is rarely possible. The more important question is, "How motivated are you to be as active as you can be, responsible for functioning as best you can, and presenting yourself to others in as healthy a manner as possible?"

A CLASSIC EXAMPLE OF HOW MOTIVATION AFFECTS PAIN

Bill was a proud, hard working husband and father of four who made a six-figure income. He was hurt on his job after three decades as a tool and die maker and was considered temporarily disabled. It became clear after a few years that Bill could not ever return to his former employment. He knew that he was likely to make only one third as much money in any other job that he might secure through vocational rehabilitation—a job that he also would not enjoy as much.

Although intensely motivated to get rid of his pain, and return to his former job, Bill was not motivated to work in any other capacity. If he were judged to be 100 percent permanently disabled, he would receive a lifetime disability income far in excess of what he would make from a new job. No one in his situation would want to work a full-time job that he did not enjoy, in pain especially, to make less money than he could by staying at home. Understandably, Bill became highly motivated to be considered legally 100 percent disabled.

Bill's almost desperate motivation for permanent disability income began to affect most of his thoughts, feelings, and behaviors. To provide support for his legal case, he became increasingly attentive to his pain and limitations, which he documented exhaustively. As we have demonstrated in earlier chapters, this increased attention actually increased his pain by increasing excitatory input from the ascending tract of the dorsal horn of the spinal cord while decreasing inhibitory input in the descending tract from the brain, i.e., it opened the pain gates wide. Of course, this escalating pain increased Bill's physical limitations. His naturally fluctuating pain levels became a source of intense focus. He continually stated that his daily pain peaks alone would prevent him from working.

Bill was the sole wage earner in the family. His wife's job was to perform all the domestic duties and to handle all the child-rearing responsibilities. Throughout Bill's treatment, his wife maintained all her responsibilities, which he still considered her role, in spite of the fact that he was no longer working. Even when she took on part-time employment, Bill refused to help around the house. He simply did not believe that it was a man's role to do domestic chores. Additionally, since he was collecting temporary disability payments, he believed he was still fulfilling his financial responsibilities. The fact that he did not have to work to get paid was irrelevant in his opinion.

As you might imagine, Bill was under intense pressure from all fronts to help his wife with domestic chores and child rearing. His initial response was to claim to be "too injured" to perform even the easiest of domestic chores. He quickly settled into lying on the couch 24/7 as his family and his life swirled around him. Since people lose about 3 percent of muscle tone per day of bed rest, he became profoundly de-conditioned, i.e., physically weak. His pain escalated further and real limitations increased.

Because Bill had little to distract himself, his attention focused on his steadily escalating pain and misery, completing a vicious cycle of spiraling pain, inactivity, and limitations. His wife began to work full time and a family member came to the home daily to care for his children. Eventually, his entire family revolved around him, his pain, and his couch. This turn of events was completely understandable and even logical under the circumstances, but unnecessary.

Though Bill would have traded his current life for his previous pain-free life in a heartbeat, he was very unmotivated to maximize his ability to be functional and productive in spite of his pain. Quite the contrary, he was very motivated to be consistently dysfunctional, even though this eventually affected his pleasurable and social activities as well. Still, he continued to pursue various interventions for pain relief.

I would like to impress you with how I helped Bill change his situation for the better, but that would be a lie. The best I could do was to ensure that he was at least aware of how and why he had created his situation and what he could choose to do about it. As of this writing, little has changed in his life and he has terminated treatment with me. The motivational issues represented in this example are surprisingly common and they occur in many guises.

FOUR MOTIVATIONAL BARRIERS TO PAIN RECOVERY

Medical doctors often consult with pain psychologists to discuss motivational issues and assess "how much this patient wants to get better." This issue is almost never discussed by medical professionals with their patients. Problems with dishonesty, noncompliance, and lack of perseverance with treatment can make a patient appear to be unmotivated to maximize their ability to manage daily responsibilities.

If a patient appears to be wrestling with severe motivational barriers to healthier functioning, the medical providers ask themselves two questions to refine their diagnosis: 1) Are the motivational barriers produced by internal needs or external reward? 2) Are these barriers conscious or unconscious? The interaction between these two possible sets of barriers to recovery creates four possible categories of motivational problems.

You could consciously create or exacerbate pain and limitations because of internal needs or external reward. Conversely, you might unconsciously create or exacerbate pain and limitations because of internal needs or external rewards. These four categories are referred to as Factitious Disorder, Malingering, primary gain, and secondary gain, respectively. It is time for me to address this minefield of political incorrectness.

The Desire to Adopt the "Sick Role"

With Factitious Disorder and Malingering, the motivational barriers are conscious and intentional. In Factitious Disorder, a patient deliberately pretends to be sick or injured to satisfy the internal need to assume the "sick" or patient role. This is a highly unusual syndrome in a typical chronic pain population, and inevitably prevents even marginally healthy social and occupational functioning. This was not a significant barrier in Bill's case.

Consciously Exaggerating Real Pain and Disability

Malingering is defined by Webster's Dictionary as, "to pretend incapacity to avoid duty or work." *The Diagnostic and Statistical Manual of Mental Disorders*, Fourth Edition (1994) describes malingering as, "the intentional production of false or grossly exaggerated physical or psychological symptoms motivated by external incentives." Whereas Factitious Disorder is always pathological, malingering may be perfectly adaptive in some situations.

Bill certainly appeared to demonstrate some intentional exaggeration of real pain complaints, but this may have been adaptive in his mind given his life situation. With people in pain, malingering rarely involves making up symptoms, but is more often a conscious exaggeration of pain or physical limitations to obtain an external reward, usually money, or attention.

If a patient has undergone three spinal surgeries and has severe chronic pain, physical weakness, limitations, and depression, she may realize accurately that she is incapable of meaningful and gainful employment. Application for Social Security Disability or other Long-Term Disability benefits is likely. Since the patient knows that she cannot work, she may consciously endorse a litany of symptoms that are greater than she actually experiences to justify a disability that she knows to be real. In this situation she would believe "the end justifies the means," and in this context, perhaps rightly so. Malingering in this situation might be dishonest, but completely adaptive from a survival perspective.

Developing Painful Symptoms through Primary Gain

Many patients would neither invent symptoms nor admit to themselves that they were exaggerating symptoms. Primary gain is the unconscious development or gross exacerbation of a physical symptom as a defense mechanism to satisfy the internal need to avoid psychological pain. It is called primary because the benefit is internal and intrinsic to the person.

The most profound example of primary gain is called conversion disorder. Real life examples include developing hysterical blindness after witnessing a horrific event, or developing hysterical paralysis in an offending limb after committing a horrific act. A well-known example in pain literature is the woman who developed stinging pain in her left cheek after learning of her husband's sexual infidelity. She described this event as "feeling like I had been slapped across the face." Primary gain is relatively infrequent in pain populations.

Worsening Pain and Disability through Secondary Gain

However, secondary gain is common in pain patients, even if the pain condition on balance is life destroying. With secondary gain, we are not referring primarily to the unconscious development of symptoms but unconscious symptom magnification to achieve an external reward.

In Bill's case, the secondary gains were disinterest in working any job other than his original one, a desire for disability income, and staunch avoidance of any domestic chores. Although some of his actions were consciously intended to achieve a reward (malingering), most of the gain was unconscious (secondary gain). Worse still, the conscious motivation to avoid domestic chores faded into the unconscious motivation to avoid specific chores at a given time. This resulted in Bill spending all day on the couch, which subsequently increased his real pain. Herein lies the tragedy inherent in all types of "gain" problems. Inevitably, they will produce increased pain, limitations, and suffering.

Other types of secondary gain can be more subtle. Chronic pain negatively affects the vast majority of marriages or partnerships. However, some spouses of people in pain are described as incredibly caring, so much so that the relationship may be described as better since the pain problem began. If a decreased ability to function results in marital improvement, this can't help but create a motivational barrier to maximal function.

You Cannot Simultaneously Seek to Justify Disability and Maximize Function

Sometimes patients are confronted with terms like malingering, secondary gain, or symptom magnification in consultations with their doctors, though it occurs more commonly in medical-legal reports or emergency room visits. Most patients feel angry, misunderstood, and persecuted as they think, "I would do anything to get rid of this pain, to get my old life back." But the real issue is, "Would you do anything to feel a little better? Would you give up some hard-won security to maybe feel a little better?"

A person may finally be accepted for Social Security Disability benefits, which provide monthly payments and Medicare health insurance. Perhaps after a year, he is feeling a little better and considering trying to return to work in some capacity. If he returns to work and fails, he may again be without Social Security payments or Medicare. This is a huge risk to take and his desire for financial security may unconsciously prompt an increased perception of disability and an unwillingness to try to return to work.

I challenge you to appreciate that you cannot pursue war and peace at the same time. The human brain is not that sophisticated. From a biochemical perspective, you cannot employ a healthy Personal Pain Paradigm that is pouring inhibitory pain signals from the brain down the descending tract of the spinal cord to minimize pain, while simultaneously focusing on pain limitations. Being compelled to attend to pain and limitations, due to your pursuit of disability, necessarily shuts down chemicals from the brain that can inhibit pain. You cannot open and close the same pain gates at the same time.

From a practical perspective, you cannot desperately pursue State Disability, Social Security Disability, private Long-Term Disability, Worker's Compensation Disability, or personal injury lawsuits, and be completely committed to demonstrating maximal function and well-being. You can't use pain to avoid unpleasant chores or other responsibilities, and remain focused on functioning at your best. This is simply not possible.

You would not show up for your Social Security hearing or personal injury trial trying to show the judge your absolute best, the healthiest you. This would be figurative suicide. Unfortunately, we have seen that if you are not consistently demonstrating maximal function and well-being, your pain and limitations will worsen as you open the pain gates wide.

Cut yourself some slack here. There are times when it is simply not in your best interests to put your best foot forward. We have discussed the importance of trying to look your best by showering, shaving, and dressing well, whether staying at home or going out. Most patients present themselves very casually when they have appointments with their pain doctor. However, many patients have noticed that on the occasions when they dress up and groom themselves as if they were going to work, the doctor may think they are feeling better because they look better. They fear he may be less willing to increase medications or provide aggressive pain treatments, such as injections. This is not always imagined. Even skilled professionals can make this mistake.

When the above issue is discussed with patients, many will think, "Well, I still want to improve my function to the maximum. I will simply choose when I want to show that maximal function." This simple sounding solution may be necessary, but cannot be completely effective. It is difficult to act and look as if you feel better than you do. It needs to become a habit, an automatic reflex. Operating at your best is an attitude and a process of structuring your day that needs to become ingrained. It is a way of living with pain, not something you can turn on and off like a light switch.

Still, it is a fact that there are many situations when it is not adaptive to function at your best. For instance, in some social situations, if you are able to act as if you feel better than you do for a little while, people may think you have recovered and begin making demands again for your time or involvement in activities that exceed your limits.

Using the information in this chapter, over the next few weeks, take an honest, hard look at your overall life situation. Be courageous and notice the times when it is not in your best interest to appear at your absolute best. How often does that happen? How important are the events when that happens? Are you involved in any situation in which you need to "prove" your disability, for legal reasons or otherwise? How much time do you spend thinking about the negative consequences of looking your best? For example, many of my worker's compensation patients are videotaped doing something that could make them look healthier than they are. Frequently, they begin to avoid doing things or leaving their home because they are afraid of the "sub rosa" videotape.

By becoming aware of your motivational challenges, you are in a better position to honestly assess your pain problem, establish your goals, make important decisions, and help your medical providers better help you.

God bless Jane, the most humorous and candid example of gain I have ever seen. We were discussing treatment options that might decrease her pain and improve her quality of life. She had been recommended for spine surgery by several highly respected and conservative spine surgeons. Jane asked me how it would affect her legal case if she recovered because of conservative treatment or surgery, i.e., would she get less money for her disability? I said that she would get less money only if her condition were significantly improved on objective tests, and if she were much more functional with much less pain and suffering. She told me that she was planning to buy a house with her settlement money, and could not afford to get any less even if it meant her condition was immensely improved. Thus, she would only consider surgery or other medical treatments that might help her recover after her case was settled.

I must confess that her honesty made me smile, and for a moment, I was dumb struck. Then I thanked her for her candor and congratulated her for establishing her priorities. She heartily agreed when I suggested that the best way we could help her was to eliminate additional treatments so that she could settle her case as quickly as possible. Her honesty with me allowed her to settle her case a year or two earlier than she would have otherwise and she loves her new home. This is important because she still hurts like hell, is nearly housebound, and refuses to pay for spine surgery out of her own pocket. Choices.

Chronic pain is an extraordinarily complex, multifaceted problem that changes every aspect of your life. In the midst of the chaos, you must try to carve out some security and stability. You can be open and honest with yourself about what that means, and what it will look like. You do not have to make apologies for the decisions you make. It is your life and your body. You get to determine what is best for you.

My real pain and limitations are worsened by any benefits that stem from my condition

Insight—I understand that whether they are conscious or unconscious, internal or external benefits will make my pain condition worse.

Commitment—I am committed to determine honestly how the four barriers to motivation may be increasing my pain and limitations and I will make changes if I so choose.

Action—In my TAAP journal, I will document any possible benefits from my pain condition, no matter how small.

Now—Even though I am desperate to feel better, I can admit that there is or was one possible benefit from my pain when: _____

26

How a Difficult Patient Appears to Doctors and Staff

You do not want to be known as a difficult, demanding, or resistant patient. It will inevitably and irrevocably compromise the quality and type of treatment that you receive. This is a fact as sure as tomorrow dawns another day. Most medical providers will deny this because it sounds so diplomatically incorrect to acknowledge that some patients might get better or different care than others. But we discussed in earlier chapters that the quality of your care is heavily influenced by your communication and relationship with your doctor. His perception of your position on the pain-suffering continuum does, and should, affect your care. The more difficult you are, the more all your providers will believe your pain is strongly shaded on the suffering side of the continuum. At a minimum, this will affect the aggressiveness of the medical treatments you will receive; as it should.

I think a caveat is in order before we proceed. You are not a difficult patient simply because you have not responded well to some treatments or because you have allergies. You are not difficult because you are assertive with doctors or staff, or because you complain when the doctor is two hours late. You are not difficult because you expect to be treated professionally and respectfully. You are not difficult because you try to direct your own care and make your own decisions. You are not difficult because you are reluctant to take medication or undergo a recommended procedure. You are not difficult because you need a little extra TLC, or a little extra time, or because your case is complicated. Pain clinics live for complicated. You are the boss of you.

You may not know that one way or another, medical patients have been receiving different qualities and types of care for thousands of years. There is an entire field of medical research called treatment disparities that evaluates how and why different groups of individuals receive different levels of medical treatment.

Usually, the most important factors are finances and medical insurance benefits. This translates into what treatments your insurance will cover, and whether or not you can make out-of-pocket payments regardless of insurance status.

However, on an individual basis, your relationship with your doctor and his staff and the credibility you have with them can strongly affect both the quality of your pain care and the type of treatments recommended. This is also something you can control. Take a Cleansing Breath and prepare yourself for the next few pages. Okay. So what does an extremely difficult patient look like?

DIFFICULT PATIENTS MAINTAIN UNREALISTIC EXPECTATIONS OF THEMSELVES AND OTHERS

Difficult patients have unrealistic expectations for their treatment outcome, which they are unwilling to change even after extensive education. No matter how long they have experienced pain, or undergone treatments, these patients believe that it is the doctor's role to provide them with a definitive diagnosis, and then to fix whatever is wrong.

Perhaps they believe the doctor's job is to provide them with whatever treatments or medications are necessary to make them comfortable. They assume that if they are not comfortable the doctor has failed and is incompetent. They may believe their doctor is solely responsible for their improvement and all they have to do is show up for their appointments. They may believe it is the doctor's responsibility to keep track of all aspects of their treatment history so they do not have to document anything.

Difficult patients often refuse to accept the chronicity of their pain problem or the importance of assuming ultimate responsibility for their treatment outcome. They may have a long history of passive, dependent behavior with strong tendencies toward the external control fallacy, believing that most of what happens to them is out of their control.

Other patients may not be as passive but perceive the body as a car, the doctor as a mechanic, and themselves as just along for the ride. They are highly unlikely to commit to self-management or to the process of developing a healthy Personal Pain Paradigm. It is much easier for them to blame others. Both types of patients may be overly encouraged in the Discovery stage of treatment and overly disillusioned during the Mapping or Building stages.

Difficult patients maintain unrealistic expectations about the process of treatment and the responsibilities of their doctor and his staff. They think it is the doctor's responsibility to make sure they set a follow-up appointment. They think the doctor should fill out all necessary medical, legal, or disability forms or write letters on his own time and for free. They think it is the doctor's job to pull information from them.

They think the doctor should remember all aspects of their case during appointments or review their chart in its entirety before appointments. They may believe that if they leave a message for the doctor to call them, he is obligated to do so. They may believe that leaving a single message for a staff member to call them back relieves them of responsibilities for appointment cancellation, following up with treatment, or notification of side effects. If they call their doctor at 5:00 p.m. on Friday because they just realized they would run out of their triplicate opioid on Saturday, they think that it is their doctor's problem.

Some of these patients are fundamentally lazy and accustomed to taking the easy way out. This can include little white lies or near constant blaming. They tend to be judgmental and feel entitled in many areas of their life. They have high performance standards for other people who are constantly falling short of their yardstick. They tend to be defensive. They are more focused on not being blamed for a problem than trying to solve it. They haven't met a doctor yet who operated a clinic as well they would.

DIFFICULT PATIENTS ARE DISHONEST AND CAUSE CONFLICT WITH STAFF

Difficult patients lie to their pain doctors, nurses, and staff. They lie about the reasons for missing, or being late for appointments. They lie about being compliant with therapies or lost medications. They lie about side effects of medications or other treatments. They lie about their symptoms. They lie about their goals and agendas, and try to manipulate the outcome they seek instead of being direct about what they want. They lie about the benefits they receive from treatment.

They lie about doing homework assigned by their providers. They say, "I will do anything to feel better," when what they really mean is, "I will come here and let you do anything you want to me, but for God's sake don't ask me to do anything." They lie about their medical and psychological histories to avoid embarrassment or to protect legal cases. A difficult patient lies about all these things and then blames the doctor for not feeling better.

Difficult patients use the rules of civil interaction and the politeness of other people as a weapon against them. They are used to lying and getting away with it.

This is such a part of their character that they are not always aware that they are lying. They may pretend to themselves that they are just exaggerating or are guilty only by error of omission. They feel completely justified in lying. Ultimately, these people are not being honest with themselves or others. They will respond defensively and with rage if they are confronted with one of their lies.

Difficult patients create a toxic clinic environment. They complain loudly in the waiting room about their pain and what the various doctors are not doing about it. They regale any other patient who will listen to their tale of woe, convinced that it is unique and worse that anyone else's. They may complain bitterly about the length of wait or the chairs.

They are inevitably unhappy with one or more staff members to whom they nearly refuse to speak because of something the employee did or said to them. They give unsolicited advice to other patients, which is unhealthy, misinformed, or otherwise negative. They have little if anything positive to say to anyone, and bring a dark cloud with them wherever they go.

Difficult patients try to create conflict between providers, between providers and staff, or between other patients and staff or doctors. They bring their young children to the office and allow them to wreak havoc with the waiting room or other patients. They expect staff to care for their children while they are in the exam room, or expect the doctor to be able to function while being terrorized by "little Johnny." They do not bring any toys or crayons for their three-year-old and when she starts acting out, they punish her loudly or pressure the staff to see the doctor immediately. When such toxic patients leave the office, staff and other patients alike breathe a sigh of relief. Of course, this is never discussed.

At the very least, these people are extremely self-absorbed and feel entitled. They may not be able to recognize how they are perceived. At worst, there appears to be a genuine malevolence in these folks that derives pleasure from other people's suffering or at least feels validated when they can create conflict. One way to feel good about yourself is to criticize others.

Difficult patients use pain as an excuse for being rude. They are frequently hostile and confrontational. They treat staff in a condescending way, barely tolerating the staff's level of alleged incompetence and communicating how different they were when they were working—back before electricity. Difficult patients never say please or thank you. They do not acknowledge or appreciate anything we do for them. Why should they? They're paying for it, aren't they?

Some of these patients are of the belief that, "It's better to be feared than liked." Simple civility is perceived as being weak. They decided long ago that you only get what you can take, that the only thing people respond to is power, demonstrated by being nasty.

DIFFICULT PATIENTS ARE NONCOMPLIANT AND MELODRAMATIC

Difficult patients are noncompliant. They are hours late for appointments and expect that they should still be seen. They miss appointments and expect their doctor to "squeeze them in tomorrow." They do not take their medications as prescribed and do not think they should have to. They attend therapy when they want to or feel like it. They are frequently "in too much pain" to comply with requests, like picking up their triplicate opioids. They do not complete homework assignments. They always have a reason why they cannot meet with the biofeedback therapist or attend pain class. They are extremely angry and defensive when they are confronted with being noncompliant. They confuse having a reason for being noncompliant with being compliant.

These patients do not believe they should have to follow the rules, usually because they are special. Part of the reason they frequently lie is because the rules do not apply to special people. They also assume that basic civility will prevent other people from confronting them about their refusal to follow the rules. Because they are accustomed to taking the easy way out, they have a history of not persevering with tasks, jobs, or relationships.

Difficult patients present themselves in the most impaired manner possible. They do not take regular pain medicine before appointments because, "I want the doctor to really be able to see my pain." They may not shower, dress reasonably, or perform basic hygiene before appointments. They are melodramatic in their presentation of pain behavior. They demand to lie down and may moan, grown or scream out during simple assessments or procedures.

They seem to have frequent crises that precipitate phone calls between appointments or after hours. They go to the Emergency Room (E.R.) frequently because of severe pain or other symptoms. They may leave the E.R. too soon because the wait is too long. For years, they may hang onto the E.R. doctor's cursory diagnosis of their underlying pain problem or his expressed concern about their outpatient medical treatment.

Such patients probably have a long history of melodrama and crisis. They may crave either the attention they get from the drama or the excitement of the crisis. Either way, they probably hate dull routine more than anything. They continually create drama in their lives, and in all likelihood, they have highly conflicted but passionate relationships.

Difficult patients specialize in creating barriers to effective treatment or progress. They are "allergic" to every medication in the world, especially antidepressants, but not usually opioids or benzodiazepines. They have violent, usually emotional, reactions to almost any injection procedure. They have horrific experiences in any hospital.

All physical therapies, including aqua therapy severely increase their pain. They will answer "Yes, but…" to almost any suggestion doctors make with a half smile on their face as they explain why that will not or cannot work for their special case. Then, they complain bitterly that no one is doing anything to help them.

These people delight in frustrating others. They are the goalies, the pitchers, the corner backs of life. They do not mind being a little miserable if it means they are special or persecuted. By focusing on what they cannot do, they are free from responsibility or risk of failure.

Difficult patients identify intensely and almost completely with the damaged patient side of themselves. They have Internet user names like RSDmary or FibroBaby. They continue to use the word *sick* to describe their condition and refer to their disease. They confuse coping badly with having a more severe medical problem. Thus, their cases are always special, usually in being the most severe or difficult cases their doctor has ever seen.

They talk about their doctors being overwhelmed by the complexity of their cases. This specialness makes them uniquely qualified to help others with the same problem. They attend support groups religiously and become actively involved in the national organizations for their diagnosis.

Often, these patients' adjustments and quality of life were marginal before their pain problem developed. They were struggling before pain onset with a history of conflicts, failures, and poor judgment. Their pain diagnosis finally medicalizes and justifies their underachievement. Embracing their condition establishes a risk-free life and allows them to surrender themselves to the fates.

ASSESSING THE DIFFICULT PATIENT IN YOU

If you do not recognize yourself in any of the previous examples, good for you. You most likely take responsibility for your health and are not a toxic patient. However, almost everyone recognizes one or two of these behaviors in themselves. People forget appointments and get frustrated sometimes. Real life can interfere with treatment. Don't sweat it. Nobody's perfect.

If you recognize several of these examples in yourself, this is a gentle reminder to treat yourself and those around you a little better. The information in this book can help you. If you identify with a dozen or more of these examples, you are on the road to becoming a difficult, demanding, resistant patient. If this chapter reads like a page from your life, you are already a difficult patient. Knock it off for your own benefit. You are receiving care that is different or worse because of the way you are presenting yourself to your medical providers.

The greater the number of difficult behaviors you endorsed, the more likely it is that you are compromising your own quality of care while making yourself and those around you more miserable than they believe is necessary. I promise you that you do not want to make your pain doctor a lot more miserable than she thinks she has to be. One way or another, it will disadvantage you.

Use the information in this book as a springboard for healthy change. This chapter is not meant as an assault, but maybe a splash of cool water on hot skin. Do you consistently act like the kind of person you want to be? Maybe not. If not, you can do better.

Being perceived as a difficult patient will affect my pain and my medical care

Insight—I understand what a difficult patient looks like.

Commitment—I am committed to not being perceived as a difficult patient.

Action—I will carefully assess difficult attitudes and behaviors throughout my medical treatment and document them in my TAAP journal.

Now—I can sheepishly acknowledge the following difficult attitudes or behaviors as revealed in this chapter: _____

_____

_____

_____

_____

_____

_____

_____

27

An Honest Discussion of Suicide and Pain

I spent several months deciding if I should write a chapter on suicide and chronic pain. I have fifteen or twenty pain books in my library and none has a chapter or even more than a page about suicide. They are dry, soulless writings that end in the pat admonition, "Just say no," as popularized by Nancy Reagan. But, my emotional response to the recent death of a patient, and my commitment to openness demanded that I proceed with this chapter. As always, I will be honest, direct, and as fair minded as possible.

Suicide is a dirty little secret in the field of chronic pain treatment. In my twenty-five-year career treating medical patients, I have lost half a dozen patients to obvious or possible suicide. If you have chronic pain, there is about a 50/50 chance that you have had a suicidal thought at some point. Most people with moderate-to-severe chronic pain have at least once entertained such a thought. The dangerousness of these thoughts varies from low risk, very passive suicidal ideation to high risk, very active suicidal ideation.

UNDERSTANDING SUICIDAL THOUGHTS

Passive suicidal thoughts are those that embrace the idea of death in some way with no real intention or specifics. In the midst of a severe pain episode, you might think to yourself, "You know, it wouldn't be so bad if I just didn't wake up tomorrow morning."

Some people say, "I'd never do anything to hurt myself but death would kind of be a relief." Patients have come in with news stories of an accidental death and said to me, "I actually felt a little jealous of that person." Over the years, I have spent many hours talking to patients about these types of passive suicidal ideations, often in the context of life feeling as if it had no meaning or purpose for them anymore.

Active suicidal ideation is more serious and attention grabbing. Here, a sense of relief at death blends into thinking of ways patients might cause their own deaths. They have considered gunshot, overdose of pills, a car crash, hanging, slashing wrists, etc. They have read books or surfed the Internet for creative and final solutions, what some have referred to as "the ultimate pain reliever."

Not surprisingly, people with active suicidal ideation are more likely to take their lives than people with only passive ideation. Conversely, some patients report feeling a sense of relief or calm simply from knowing how they would kill themselves if they ever made that decision. Some patients report this helps them feel more in control of the whole process of life, death, and pain. I am not suggesting that it is healthy to decide how you would take your life, only observing that a few patients have reported feeling calmer after doing so.

Other patients have taken this one scary step further and "prepared" the means they would employ. Some have scouted out the cliffs they would drive over. Perhaps like Mel Gibson in the movie *Lethal Weapon*, they may have a gun and a special bullet. One patient carried around a vile of a few hundred ground-up Elavil for over a year, in case he was ever "pushed over the edge." Repeated attempts to convince him to discard the vial were unsuccessful, although he eventually discarded it on his own after his depression and suffering had abated somewhat.

The next type of active suicidal ideation is the "cry for help" acting out—people who are actively suicidal and make a gesture but do not intend to kill themselves. These people cut their wrists a little, call the police from the top of a cliff, or call a friend to tell them that they are overdosing. They may feel so desperate and alone that this seems like their only option for asking for help. Some people try to convince their support system that they really are in trouble by hurting themselves, in a non-lethal way.

We can feel compassion for people who are so desperate that they have felt that this was the only way to obtain help. Sometimes, their cries for help will result in unintended deaths, which is a profound tragedy. Certainly, these patients need the very best resources we have, both psycho-therapeutically and pharmacologically.

TYPES OF SUICIDAL BEHAVIORS

Two types of suicidal thinking that are reflected in someone's behavior can lead to death. The first type is the patient who does not deliberately intend to kill himself, but who does something that risks death. This person has a severe pain episode and takes a lot of extra, but nonlethal, pain medication to help him sleep. Maybe he mixes it with alcohol. He falls asleep, but in a few hours wakes up, still in pain, and takes more medication. He may repeat this cycle several times. On occasion, this person falls asleep and never wakes up. This behavior is driven by pain, frustration, and desperation.

Usually, the person is not consciously trying to kill himself. He just wants to hurt less, though in his heart, he knows he is taking a real risk. Many patients have done this without fatal consequences. It is often a matter of blind luck that it is not fatal. I have worked with several patients who "slept" for twenty-four to seventy-two hours before waking up from a medication overdose, perhaps their sleep more accurately being described as near coma.

The final level of active suicidal ideation is the completely deliberate and lethal suicide attempt that will result in death, barring miraculous interference. I'm not talking about the patient who takes 150 pills, and calls a friend. Instead, he takes 150 Schedule 2 pills, drinks a fifth of scotch, and falls asleep alone. Or, he puts a loaded gun in his mouth and pulls the trigger. Or, he drives off a cliff at sixty miles an hour. Only blind luck and random chance (or God, if you believe) can save his life.

People who seriously attempt suicide are not necessarily more depressed or otherwise more distressed than all the depressed people who did not try to kill themselves. However, people who attempt suicide appear to be more hopeless than those who do not. From a treatment perspective, increasing depression is not necessarily associated with a greater likelihood of a suicide attempt, but increasing hopelessness is. Thus, hopelessness is the intersection between chronic pain and suicide.

Keep in mind that suicidal thoughts are not the enemy. They do not mean you are crazy, or bizarre. Suicidal thoughts cannot kill you, only behavior can. Suicidal thoughts are scary because they symbolize the fact that your psychological resources are being taxed beyond their limit. These thoughts may mean that your current hierarchy of coping strategies, the path you are on now, is not adequate for the demands you are facing. This is important information for you.

People in pain can suffer devastating losses. You may lose homes, marriages, jobs, the custody of your children, financial security, friends, work colleagues, self-esteem, your identity, a sense of purpose, pleasurable activities, or sexual enjoyment. You can be crippled by anxiety over future potential losses or worsening pain and quality of life.

Beyond the catastrophic loss and fear is the pain itself—angry, punishing, excruciating, and exhausting. I believe that coping with chronic pain and the death of a child are the two most difficult events people face in the normal course of life—in many cases, more difficult than dying of illness or old age.

As you deal with the horror that can be chronic pain, it is not aberrant to consider death as an alternative. I have lost patients to suicide and dropped to my knees sobbing with my head in my hands when I was informed. With others, I have been comfortable, whispered good-bye in my prayers, and wished them a good journey and some peace. Every person is unique and each person's reason for choosing "not to be" is unique.

ACKNOWLEDGING THE CONCEPT OF RATIONAL SUICIDE

I believe that people have the right to decide what they will do with their own bodies and this includes the choice to live or die. I think that each of us has the right to decide the minimal, acceptable quality of life we require to warrant continuing to live. I would argue that people have the right to determine for themselves the relative hopelessness of their situation.

I fully respect a person's right to decide whether to live or die. In some cases, I believe in what is referred to as rational suicide and I am far more likely after this type of death to feel comfortable and wish this person "Godspeed."

I defend your right to take your life under any circumstances. But, to consider it rational, I use my own standards of common sense and thirty years of education and experience in medical psychology. This chapter has forced me to crystallize the four criteria I use for rational suicide. The criteria, that if met, usually results in my feeling somehow comfortable with the decision my patient made to die. My purpose in listing them here is not meant to give you permission to kill yourself if you fulfill the criteria, but rather to give you hope if you do not.

Criteria for Rational Suicide

First and most importantly, your current life situation must be very, very bad. The combination of circumstances must be so horrific that you would rather be dead than continue to live. How bad life must be before you can rationally consider taking your life is an individual decision, and each person makes this decision for different reasons, with different levels and types of emotional and physical pain.

I have worked with terminally ill patients who have stated that when they reached the point that they were incapable of caring for themselves for the most basic needs, e.g., feeding, bathroom, and bathing, they no longer wished to live. Although I might not feel the same way, I can understand this and it passes the common sense test. The truth is that most people who make the decision when to commit suicide before the time comes, do not act upon it when the time comes.

This is in contrast to the patient who wanted to die if she could no longer run comfortably. Or, the patient who wanted to kill herself, because she could not ice skate anymore. Some patients want to die because they cannot work or spend time with their children as they once did. Some patients have wanted to kill themselves because they thought they would lose their homes and be forced to move into apartments.

I treated a member of a motorcycle club who wanted to die because he could no longer ride a motorcycle. He had to travel by "cage," i.e., car. We know there are billions of people who live happy and productive lives, without engaging in any of the above activities, thereby making the task of these people to adjust to their limitations and try to live productive lives, not to commit suicide. They fail the common sense test.

You have learned that you have tremendous control over the suffering you experience because of terrible events in your life. Simply choosing not to exercise control over your own suffering cannot produce a rational suicide. Your situation must be so horrific that coping with it as well as anyone reasonably could, would not produce a quality of life that you believe is good enough for you to want to continue to live. You cannot know this until you are coping about as well as anyone could under similar circumstances.

The second criteria for rational suicide is that there is no possibility that your situation will improve in the future. This is not about hope exactly, but a realistic, accurate assessment of the likelihood that things will change. Physical conditions that could fit this description include paraplegia and quadriplegia, terminal illness, long-term stroke, and severe neuropathies. Psychological conditions may include certain severe mental illnesses and catastrophic losses from which there is no return.

I remember a frail, elderly patient with severe pain whose loving wife of sixty-two years had died six months earlier. He was still mentally alert and vibrant. He looked me in the eye and said, "I'm tired. I'm hurting. I miss my other half. It's time for me to go home." He died in his sleep a few weeks later with a lot of extra medication in his system. I wished him a warm homecoming.

The third criteria for rational suicide is that you have done everything feasible to try to improve your situation. Remember that chronic pain is a combination of sensation and suffering, the latter defined as thoughts, feelings, and behaviors. For pain and the sequelae to justify a rational suicide, you need to have given the medical system and hundreds of self-management strategies a fair chance, including those listed in this book or other pain books. A fair chance means not just reading a pain book or listening to a pain psychologist, but spending a year or so diligently practicing the strategies and techniques comprising your Personal Pain Paradigm—walking the walk. You cannot just decide that these things will not help because we know that they can. You need to have lived them for a time and then be able to say, "It's just not good enough."

Rational suicide implies that your suffering is so aversive *in the present* that you do not choose to continue living. It must be almost inevitably the same or worse *in the future* and out of your control. Finally, you must have done everything reasonable *in the past* to improve your situation or reduce your suffering. Then, you can know that the misery of your current situation is irrevocable.

I have conducted thousands of sessions with patients who have declined to try a pain-relieving or coping strategy simply because they did not want to, usually because they were too lazy. It fell outside of their emotional comfort zone. They refused to attend pain class, stating, "I'm just not a group person, doc." They refused to try exercising because, "You know doc, I've just never been an exerciser." They refused to tell their doctor what's really going on because, "He should know what questions to ask." They say, "I've never had to ask for help before, and I'm not gonna start now." Or, "Nuthin' personal doc, but I don't put much stock in psychology."

Again, statements like those above usually mean, "I will lie here and let you do anything you want to me, but I won't put out the effort to help myself." If you haven't done everything you can to help yourself, your suicide cannot be rational.

The fourth and final criterion for rational suicide is that it must be consistent with your basic morals, values, goals, and spiritual sense of meaning and purpose.

Moreover, rational suicide should be consistent with the common sense test of morality, values, and goals. I do not believe that it is inherently immoral to kill oneself. But, you may believe that it is immoral, perhaps because, "Only God has the right to decide life or death." In this context, you must evaluate your suicidal thoughts from the perspective of your beliefs. Your own personal integrity should make you decide not to take your life, or you need to change your belief that suicide is immoral.

It is an industry standard in the field of psychotherapy that if someone is seriously considering suicide, you should talk about the pain their loved ones will feel—use it as a weapon against their suicide. We are taught to give patients the message, "Don't kill yourself because of what it will do to your family and friends." I have a problem with that, two actually. First, other people do not hold the mortgage on your soul. They do not get to decide whether you live or die and they are responsible for how they deal with your death. They are responsible for their own thoughts, feelings, and behaviors. Your life is fully yours to control, as their lives are theirs to control.

Second, if the main reason you stay alive miserably is because of how your death would affect others, then you get to blame them for your misery. And you will. I have seen people decide not to kill themselves because of family or friends and then spend many years being a bitter, toxic influence on their supposed loved ones. This is a terrible thing to do to the people you say you love, perhaps worse than taking your life.

Rational suicide means taking all of life's benefits and costs into account, as they are consistent with your values and common sense or basic decency. Let's say a man loses his job and his mistress in the same day, so he decides to check out of Hotel Life. He leaves behind a stay-at-home wife and three children, no savings, no home equity, and no life insurance. Not only is this not rational, but it seems immoral to me—not because he is taking his life, but because he is completely abdicating his moral responsibility to his family. This situation differs dramatically from a man with severe or terminal pain whose adult children are financially secure if he dies.

If you have small children, your suicide would have devastating consequences on them. Research has consistently shown that children and families are even more affected by suicide than by accidental death or murder. There is a stigma and even a sense of blame associated with suicide that can affect multiple generations of family members. Although the impact on family and children should be a factor in your decision, it should not be the sole driving force in your decision. Your children also do not hold a mortgage on your soul. On the other hand, common sense dictates that you have a moral duty, within reasonable parameters, to see that they are mentally and physically healthy and financially secure.

My personal mission statement contains eight fundamental values or goals. Three of these values reference other people and my passionate commitment to improving the life of my nuclear and global family. For me, suicide born of personal misery would not be consistent with these three values. I would need to assess whether suicide was consistent with the other five values in the context of my current situation with a higher priority than the three family values.

Caveats about Rational Suicide

Suicidal thoughts and actions are extremely powerful and frightening, both for the suicidal person and anyone dealing with that person. Thus, suicidal statements and actions tend to get immediate and dramatic attention from one's support system and health professionals. For people who are characteristically attention seeking, melodramatic, and manipulative, a suicidal gesture can be the most effective way of getting attention.

For patients with borderline, histrionic, or narcissistic personality disorders, a suicide attempt is just a more dramatic example of "same old, same old." These patients have no intention of taking their lives or even risking it. They are trading on the pain of those who are genuinely suicidal to manipulate the people around them.

Early in my career, I remember rushing to the hospital for a pain patient following a call from her spouse telling me that she had attempted suicide by medication overdose. As my patient was being wheeled into the emergency room on a gurney, she was talking about her suicide attempt; how her spouse had saved her; and blaming her insurance company for not authorizing a certain treatment. I questioned her and discovered that her suicide attempt consisted of swallowing three Vicodin, two Flexeril, and two Xanax. Considering her tolerance from her copious regular medications, this was hardly enough to make her a little tired, and she knew that. However, it did capture the attention of all her family and friends, the medical-legal system of which she was a part and a couple dozen medical and mental health professionals for a week. I felt slimed. It is an abomination to do that to family, friends, or people trying to help you.

Suicide is the only pain-related decision from which there is no second chance. The best possible outcome of suicidal thoughts is that you analyze the relative advantages and disadvantages of suicide in a logical manner and decide you want to live. You realize that you have not done everything you can to alleviate your suffering, and you commit to living as healthily and happily as possible.

If you have not been treated in a multi-disciplinary pain setting for a year with a pain physician and pain psychologist, there is about a 90 percent chance that you are suffering more than is necessary. Therefore, it is essentially impossible for you to commit rational suicide. Even if you have received intensive treatment, you are suffering more than you need to if you have not committed to practicing the self-management techniques in this or another book for at least a year.

If you are suicidal, talk to someone about it. You do not have to go through those thoughts alone. Such thoughts cannot hurt you. Only you can hurt you. But you can help yourself, too.

Death is not the ultimate pain reliever—a purposeful life is

Insight—I understand the concept of rational suicide.

Commitment—I am committed to being rational about life and death decisions consistent with my own moral beliefs.

Action—I will carefully assess my life situation in terms of the criteria listed above. If I do not fulfill the criteria for rational suicide, I will document that in my TAAP journal and use it as a tool for hope during the dark times.

Now—If I do seem to fulfill the criteria, I will document that in pencil in my TAAP journal and talk to at least one friend and one mental health professional as soon as possible to get some additional and more objective feedback. If I subsequently decide that I do not fulfill the criteria, I will erase what I have written in pencil and document in pen why I do not fulfill the criteria.

28

Comfort for Severe Pain Episodes

People with chronic pain are more likely to commit suicide, accidentally or on purpose, when their pain is most severe. Coping with the periods when you hurt the worst is exhausting and miserable. Times of severe pain tax your emotional and coping resources to the breaking point and beyond. We have discussed the fact that pain varies by the minute, the day, and the season. Periods of severe pain are inevitable, and it is important to have a plan for dealing with them, in advance of their occurrence.

HOW TO CONCEPTUALIZE PERIODS OF SEVERE PAIN

There are two strategies for coping with severe pain. Mental and attitudinal approaches are referred to as reframing while the physical and behavioral approaches are considered comfort measures. The core attitudinal coping strategy for severe pain lies in conceptualizing severe pain as an episode, like a situational comedy on television. It has a beginning, middle, and an end. It always has an end.

Part of coping with severe pain means dealing with all the fears associated with it. Will this severe pain go away? Does this mean I am injured worse than I was before? Do I need to go to the emergency room? Can I do something to make the pain go away?

Begin by talking yourself down. The panic and rage you may feel are probably driven by some cognitive distortions or automatic negative thoughts. You can combat these and work yourself down with some positive statements, such as, "This is just a severe pain episode. I did not re-injure myself. This pain will go away soon. It always goes away. It will this time. I just need to cope right now. I can just be quiet for a while and rest. I just have to deal with it now. I only have to deal with this pain for the next three minutes."

It can be helpful to give your pain a powerful image or an overarching concept. There are three approaches to imagining a severe pain episode that can assist you not only in coping with your pain but containing it.

Imagine Your Pain as a Storm

The first approach is to imagine your pain as a storm, perhaps as follows:

The sun slips behind dark clouds. The wind picks up and the water drops begin. Distant thunder booms and jagged flashes of lightning herald fire and the smell of ozone. The wind blows a driving, horizontal rain like needles. Crashing explosions rend the earth in brilliant flashes of light. Trees are toppled or bowed down to the fury of nature. Time stops. Then, lightening fades and thunder becomes the throb of distant cannons. The wind releases and the rain softens and fades away. The sky lightens and patches of daylight peek through the clouds. The sound of birds chirping is heard once again. The earth is shaken but unharmed. Just like you after a severe pain episode.

Imagine Your Pain as an Enemy

Another image that can help you cope with severe pain is by perceiving pain as an enemy. This concept can allow you to use anger in a productive manner. I imagine my pain as a laughing, red, monkey-like devil complete with pitchfork. Your pain enemy is trying to make you do unhealthy things, such as stay on the couch, yell at the kids, take way too much medicine, or go to the emergency room. You can let yourself be angry by saying, "I won't let my enemy win. I won't do unhealthy things. I win the battle if I only do healthy things to get through this, and I can do healthy things."

In the same way that severe pain episodes have a beginning, middle, and end, so too must your anger. I have treated a number of patients who, when discussing anger as a coping mechanism for pain, have said, "I'm really good at this one, doc. I'm angry all the time."

Although anger is a common response to pain, chronic anger is never healthy. However, you can use episodes of anger constructively by refusing to lose the healthy coping battle with severe pain episodes.

Imagine Your Pain as a Teacher

The final type of image to help you cope with severe pain episodes is pain as a teacher. I call this the Zen of pain coping. You can imagine severe pain as a wise teacher that knows all and can share helpful information with you at two levels. First, you can try comfort strategies that have worked for you in the past. You can vary them as you choose. Or, you can be creative and try new strategies that you have learned in this book, from other people in pain, or from any other source.

Second, you can explore the possible triggers for this severe pain episode. What might have happened that caused or contributed to this episode? It might include weather, a slight stumble, or a sleepless night. How might you have contributed to this increased pain? Did you overdo or pace poorly? Did you let yourself run out of medicine? Did you exercise too much or too hard? Did you spend too much time on the couch the past day or week?

Conceiving of severe pain as a teacher is a great way to learn coping strategies. Focusing on how you might have caused the episode may be most helpful after the intense pain has faded somewhat. You might just get angrier with yourself and more discouraged if you place responsibility or blame in the throes of your misery. If you do identify triggers that you could have prevented, vow not to do that again. Give yourself permission to learn something positive from this pain episode. When it blessedly ends, act on your commitment and make any necessary changes to prevent another avoidable, severe pain episode.

Comfort Measures for Decreasing Severe Pain Episodes

Comfort coping refers to the things you do or let others do for you to decrease severe pain and to cope better. Comfort coping includes both passive and active strategies. Passive strategies are those things either that are done to you or that compel you to be inactive.

First is resting. Some patients with spine pain benefit by lying on their backs on the ground with their legs (from the back of the knee to the foot) up on a chair to form a 90-degree angle. This is called the neutral spine position, as it eliminates the natural curvature or lordosis of the spine. You might try receiving a massage, even a very light one. Some people benefit from acupuncture or acupressure. You could receive a session of passive physical therapy with heat or ultrasound, even if you had to pay for it.

At home, you could try heating pads, hot showers, or heating creams like Ben Gay. You might try ice wraps or cold compresses. Many people benefit the most by alternating heat and cold. You might ask your doctor for a prescription anesthetic cream. You can take extra medication as your doctor allows, most commonly opioids or muscle relaxants.

Passive distraction strategies may be helpful, such as television or listening to music. You may have available at your home a transcutaneous nerve stimulator (TENS) unit that can temporarily block pain signals. You might try an H Wave home unit that provides a type of treatment similar to ultrasound.

Active strategies are those behaviors you perform to ease your pain that involve directed activity. For instance, you might try massaging painful areas yourself, perhaps in conjunction with heat or anesthetic cream. You might try gentle, slow stretching, perhaps combined with heat, massage, or anesthetic cream. Relaxation techniques should always be employed, especially breathing, and progressive muscle relaxation. The Quick Release is an excellent relaxation technique for severe pain episodes.

Active distraction is also important and can involve phone calls, visits from friends, hobbies, playing Scrabble, or video games. You may try the STAR and STIM techniques. Go for a short walk, perhaps in a nature setting. Stay away from stimulants or overdoing. Be creative. Do not be afraid to try something new. Document in your TAAP journal all the comfort strategies that you have tried as part of your Personal Pain Paradigm.

Stay in the moment when coping with severe pain episodes. Usually, it is the fear that the severe pain episode will not go away, or not soon enough, that compels people to do unhealthy or unhelpful things. Telling yourself "I cannot take this pain all night" may send you to the emergency room. Thinking to yourself, "I couldn't stand it if this pain lasted all weekend" may result in a 5:00 p.m., Friday night call to your doctor, the bane of all pain clinics.

You do not have to deal with this pain tonight, or tomorrow, or the next day. You only have to deal with it during the next three minutes. Ask yourself, "What would I do if I only had to deal with this pain for a few minutes?" Conversely, ask, "What wouldn't I do if this pain only lasted a few minutes?"

With a severe pain episode, all you should be dealing with is the present moment. Give yourself permission to let future demands or concerns fade away. Your life purpose lives in how you handle the next three minutes.

I can learn to cope better with severe pain episodes

Insight—I understand the concept of a severe pain episode.

Commitment—Since severe pain episodes are common with chronic pain, I am committed to learning to master them more effectively.

Action—I will practice reframing strategies using storm, enemy, and teacher images, and practice all the comfort techniques I can discover or create.

Now—I believe that the _____ reframing technique will work best for me and that my most effective comfort techniques for severe pain episodes are:_____

_____

_____

_____

_____

_____

_____

_____

_____

29

I Should Be Hopeful and Optimistic

You may remember that Rhia was a 48-year-old, Welsh, divorced female with a thirteen-year history of chronic, severe, low back pain who was status post three lumbar surgeries including spinal fusion from L3-S1 with hardware and iliac crest grafting. She lived in her own apartment but had 24-hour, in-home, nursing care. She had spent twenty-three hours of each day in bed for the past year. She was profoundly depressed and had been admitted to a psychiatric facility twice in the past year for suicide attempts. She was taking eleven medications, including psychotropics and twenty Vicodin a day. She was a recovering alcoholic with seventeen years of sobriety but smoked two packs a day. She had no friends, and she was estranged from her adult children.

Rhia would be able to proceed through our pain program in her current condition only if we provided her with significant pain relief as we worked on increasing her activity level. Since her in-home care provider was her only social contact, we also had to assure her that she would not lose her care provider unless she made dramatic progress and had developed a social network. She moved with her care provider into a hospital-based residence near the pain clinic that had been established for out-of-town patients and family.

During Rhia's first week in treatment, she received heat, ultrasound, and daily massage treatments in the morning, biofeedback, and various classes in the early afternoon, and finished with a hot tub treatment toward late afternoon. She and her care provider brought all of her Vicodin, Percocet, Darvon, etc., into the office, and she was switched to MS Contin, a long-acting opioid in a slightly higher dose than her Vicodin.

She was taking four benzodiazepine type medications that we combined into one, Valium, that she took three times daily. She remained angry, frustrated, and suicidal. She made severe demands on the staff and would not tolerate the slightest inconveniences. She complained bitterly about her pain, and made it clear to us that her pain was worse than any other patient's pain.

During the second week of treatment, Rhia admitted to having had a long history of panic attacks for which she had been taking anxiolytics for years. She was placed on a tricyclic antidepressant, amitriptyline, at bedtime to help her sleep. We titrated her dose of Prozac to 80 mgs.

She remained severely hostile, depressed, and anxious. From her perspective, she was being forced by the insurance company to participate in our program. We continued the passive therapy modalities but added aqua therapy to her afternoon hot tub regimen. She graduated from a gurney to a wheelchair, but was enraged, claiming that we were pushing her too fast.

Over the next two weeks, Rhia completed her daily behavioral and psychology classes. We then increased the amitriptyline at bedtime and eliminated one of her daily tabs of Valium. She began treatment with the anticonvulsant Neurontin that was gradually titrated. In individual behavioral treatment, we were working on her panic attacks with in vitro desensitization by having her imagine her feared stimuli, in her case crowds, and maintaining relaxation. She began attending appointments using a walker. She continued to complain severely but began to smile occasionally at the office. She was staying out of bed for up to eight hours a day.

During the four weeks after that, Rhia began land-based physical therapy three times per week, and enrolled in aqua exercise classes at the same pool she had been using for aqua therapy. Passive physical therapy ended except for twice-weekly massages. She complained of increased pain from the land-based, active physical therapy combined with being up over eight hours per day.

We increased Rhia's dose of MS Contin from 60 mgs three times per day to 80 mgs three times per day. We decreased her Valium to one tablet a day. Her anxiety decreased considerably and her sleep improved. Her anger, frustration, and sense of persecution reached a plateau.

She agreed to release her caretaker for the eight bedtime hours. Twice weekly, I took her to a nearby mall where we ate lunch and she was re-integrated into being among crowds. Her attitude was much softer and less angry during these lunches, which generalized to a global improvement in attitude by the end of this four-week period. Finally, she acknowledged that her pain had improved.

Rhia seemed on the road to recovery and was feeling pretty good about herself. By all accounts, she was happier and functioning better. They say life is always good before a fall.

In the ninth week, she began to miss appointments and at times, her speech was slurred. We discovered at week's end that she had resumed drinking after seventeen years of sobriety. All she could tell us was that she felt healthier than she had in ten years and she had no reason to drink.

I believed that she was afraid of all the dramatic changes that were happening to her and the increasing expectations that her progress was creating. She had not been responsible for herself at even a basic level for almost a decade, and she was terrified by the thought of being independent. On the surface, she practiced the strategy of "the best defense is a good offense" and resumed being hostile, blaming, and difficult.

We made sobriety from alcohol a requirement for Rhia's continued participation in the program. She agreed to take Antabuse after much discussion and anger. For the next month, she took Antabuse daily including twice a week while at our office. By that time, she ambulated with a walker, and was out of bed twelve of her sixteen waking hours. She had begun paying her own bills. She had developed several friendships with other patients at the residence and with the in-house resident manager. She agreed to release her in-home caretaker for another eight-hour shift, leaving her with eight hours of care. She was much less difficult and angry at the end of the month and seemed happier again. She started a genealogy project to explore her Welsh heritage, which had always been very important to her.

Rhia was again trying to work some of the steps in her Alcoholics Anonymous program and decided to try to re-establish contact with her estranged adult children, initially her daughter. The conversation went badly and her daughter declined to resume a relationship. Rhia was devastated by the reality that she would probably never have a relationship with her daughter.

In the weeks that followed, Rhia began abusing her narcotic pain medicine, and was discovered having scripts from another doctor. Although she remained sober from alcohol, her behavior deteriorated and she again became, angry, blaming, anxious, and severely depressed with resumption of suicidal ideation. She took a potentially lethal overdose of her medication, and was admitted to the hospital.

Rhia spent three days on an acute care medical floor, and was then transferred to the psychiatric unit. In consultation with a psychiatrist, the decision was made to detox her from all medications except her antidepressants and anticonvulsant. She surrendered all her medications. She became surprisingly acquiescent to these changes but was emotionally flat. Perhaps she had truly given up on herself. I had hospitalized hundreds of patients psychiatrically, but with her symptoms and terrible life situation, I, too, was not feeling very hopeful. Western medicine just seemed inadequate.

On the afternoon that Rhia was scheduled to return home from the hospital, I stopped off at a new age bookstore looking for a gift for her since she was a believer in all things occult, e.g., astrology, numerology, and signs. She was an aging hippy and had once earned a living reading tarot cards. The store was full of dark wood and earthy smells. I wandered past crystals, incense, herbs, and stones, into the section with books about witchcraft and fairy tales.

I leafed through a book of ancient Welsh fairy tales and stopped short when I saw the title, *Rhiannon's Sorrow*. Rhia's name was short for Rhiannon. Her proud, Welsh parents had given her the name descended from this character in Welsh lore whether they knew it or not. I read the story, and felt overcome with poignancy and hope. I went home, typed it, had it framed at a store while I waited, and gift-wrapped it in my car at the hospital.

When I got to Rhia's room, I said that I was stopping by to give her a present for having worked so hard the past four months, and to encourage her that she would find some happiness and purpose again. She unwrapped the gift and began reading about her namesake (Appendix). She must have read it more than once. At some point, her eyes welled up with tears, her chest heaved, and she started to cry. Eventually, she rested her forehead on the picture frame with her eyes closed and stayed that way. Minutes passed and the only sound was the ticking of the wall clock. Then she looked up at me and said, "I didn't know." We hugged hard and healthily. I told her I would see her at the clinic the next day, and I left.

Rhia seemed different after that. She made slow, steady progress. She still had some ups and downs but they were less catastrophic. She graduated from a walker to a cane. She let go of her care provider for the final eight-hour shift, but maintained a housekeeper for four hours a week. She smiled and laughed some. She began to socialize more and even developed a few friendships. She was able to resume a relationship with her son and her grandchildren. When it was time for her to leave the hospital residence, she actually obtained employment as a resident apartment manager.

Seven months into Rhia's treatment, additional discs in her spine collapsed causing severe pain. She had an indwelling narcotic pump implanted, and for her this was another turning point. She obtained excellent pain relief, walked completely upright for the first time, and was able to be active fourteen of sixteen waking hours. She was sober and remained off all oral medications except for Prozac, Elavil, and Neurontin. She said her self-esteem was higher than at any point in her life. She was happy more days than not.

One year after her first appointment, I conducted an exit interview since she was officially entering the maintenance phase of treatment and we would only be meeting every four to six weeks. We had been through a lot together and shared a relationship born of battles lost and won. Though we had excellent rapport by now, as she was getting ready to leave, I asked her what had changed? What was different? If she had only one wish, what would it be? For the first time that day, she showed an extra spark (along with a distant memory). She pulled herself up in her chair, looked me straight in the eyes, and said, "I want to live."

◆   ◆   ◆

Hope is the anti-suicide feeling. Hope is the existential angst conqueror. Hope is your brain's way of saying, "Life still has value, and so do I."

Webster's Dictionary defines the verb *hope* as, "to cherish a desire with anticipation." Specifically, it is the feeling associated with the belief that a desired goal <u>can</u> be achieved. It is the belief that life can change in a clearly defined way for the better. You might say, "I hope there is peace in the world."

Webster's defines the noun *hope* as, "desire accompanied by expectation of or belief in fulfillment." Here, hope includes an expectation or a confidence that the goal <u>will</u> be achieved, that life will change for the better. You might say," I am hopeful I will have less pain."

Optimism is a term that combines Latin roots meaning, "best power." It is defined as "an inclination to put the most favorable construction upon actions and events, or to anticipate the best possible outcome." An optimist sees the glass as half full and ready to hold even more water. She may tend to see the goodness in herself and others more than the badness. Her personality predisposes her to perceive the present and the future in generally positive ways. She believes in a good future.

HOW TO MAINTAIN HOPE AND OPTIMISM WITH CHRONIC PAIN

Hope and optimism are life-affirming feelings associated with certain perceptions or beliefs. What makes you believe that your life and your pain can get better? What makes you believe that your life and your pain will get better? What makes you believe that life can still have meaning while struggling against the misery and suffering of pain? The simple answer is to live the first twenty-eight chapters of this book for a year. But life is not so simple.

The most valuable insight into pain is the knowledge that pain and function are opposite sides of the same coin. The amount of pain you experience is dependent on your level of activity. In the short term, if you artificially increase your activity, your pain will increase somewhat. In the short term, if you rest a little, your pain will probably decrease.

The above insight means that you can decrease pain in either of two ways. You can have decreased pain with the same amount of activity. Conversely, you can increase your activity without the expected increase in pain. Perhaps, you reach the point where cooking dinner does not increase your pain like it did for two straight years. That is a pain decrease. Of course, decreased pain with increased activity is the best of both worlds.

This insight creates two possibilities for having less pain and feeling better, two opportunities for hope, two chances to believe that your life and your pain can get better. You can use some or all of the strategies in this book for decreasing pain. You can try the strategies for increasing activity without increasing pain. You can try both types of strategies with a greater likelihood that you will achieve nirvana, increasing activity with steadily decreasing pain. You can know that many thousands of people have committed to these strategies and felt better with improved quality of life.

THE POWER OF SCIENCE IN PAIN RELIEF

You can believe in the power of science. Billions of dollars are spent on chronic pain research every year. We are learning so much about pain transmission and pain relief. Spinal cord stimulators and narcotic pumps are the stuff of science fiction, but are available today. There is research on super powerful opioids that more closely mirror endorphins and enkephalins. One research line is working on developing chemicals that block chronic pain but not acute pain because they travel different routes and use different if overlapping nerve fibers.

New techniques are being developed for treating muscular pain, from stimulating devices to injections to specific medications. New generation neuropathic pain medications are being explored, as well as deep brain surgical procedures that can block pain altogether. For spine pain, there are new surgical treatments becoming available that were almost unthinkable a few decades ago.

Every year, new treatments for chronic pain are introduced. You can be assured that, in the United States, as the baby boomers age and hurt more, a larger percentage of funds from the federal government and private industry will be spent to find solutions for chronic pain. This is real and it is happening now.

THE POWER OF PRACTICING THE ABCS OF PAIN RELIEF AND TREATMENT

The best predictor of future behavior is past behavior. The best way for you to believe that future pain and functioning will improve is to create a history of your own improvement. Commit to refining and enhancing your Personal Pain Paradigm. Use it as you might a wise, old friend to proceed with your journey toward personal growth, decreased pain, and improved function.

You have learned how your doctors can best help you through the eleven-step hierarchy of pain treatments. You understand the notion of multifactoral pain, and now you know how to negotiate better care from your doctors. You were taught the four stages of pain treatment, and you learned how to make the best progress though them. You learned how to maximize the benefits of medications and physical therapies.

You have learned how you can best help you. You can minimize pain behaviors and increase physical activity. You know how to exercise and recondition strength, flexibility, and endurance without increasing pain. You were taught strategies for pacing and limit setting. You learned the mechanics of healthy movement and the red, yellow, and green zones. You explored active listening skills and strategies for improving social activity. You discovered the Pleasure Pyramid for enjoyable activity and the Mastery Map for Productive Activity. You learned how to manage thoughts and feelings more effectively to reduce suffering. You were taught how to make important changes in your lifestyle and the benefits of nutritional supplements in your global health and pain paradigm. You learned how to better manage severe pain episodes.

You have learned how you can best help your doctor help you. You can identify and conquer motivational challenges to maximize activity and function. You assessed difficult behaviors that may affect the medical aggressiveness of your doctor's treatment. You understand the importance of compliance with treatments and maintenance of credibility with your doctor.

You can document all of these struggles and victories in your TAAP journal. You will be building confidence that you can continue to improve because you will have a history of your progress. You can review your Personal Pain Paradigm whenever you feel discouraged, and know that you can conquer the challenges along the road to pain relief.

I created the PPP Assessment to propel you forward and to maintain a steady course toward pain relief. It is based upon the principles in this book, and it consists of 170 True-False statements that you can complete in about fifteen minutes. It is computer scored, and generates a twenty-to-thirty page report that reveals the thirty-one most important elements specific to your emerging Personal Pain Paradigm. You also find your place on the Pain vs. Suffering continuum, and you learn the probability that medical or behavioral interventions will be successful.

Any pain book is limited by the difficulty in providing recommendations that are uniquely applicable to the individual reader. This advice requires a comprehensive, individual assessment, such as from the PPP Assessment. The report is presented as if I were your pain psychologist giving you detailed feedback after an office assessment. You are given honest, incisive counsel to refine your Personal Pain Paradigm, from which you can draw strength, and discover the specific changes necessary to produce the greatest pain relief. All you have to do is respond to the statements honestly.

You can complete the PPP Assessment and acquire your report at www.MyPainReliefDoc.com, or by writing to Dr. Tim Sams, c/o PACE, Inc., P.O. Box 6599, Irvine, CA, 92616. Or, you can call my toll-free number, 877-545-7272, for more information.

You have learned that pain includes sensation, thoughts, feelings, and behaviors, all of which affect each other. You know in your heart that you can affect your thoughts, feelings, and behaviors. This establishes as a certainty that you can affect your pain. You absolutely, positively can hurt less. You can speed inhibitory chemicals down the dorsal horn of your spinal cord and vigorously close those pain gates. But, will you do the things that you know are necessary to hurt less? Are pain relief and increased function important enough for you to take action? Only you can answer those questions. Only you know if the reward is worth the effort. But, therein lies hope—your improvement determined solely by your own motivation to feel better—pain relief by choice.

A new day dawns with promise in your quest for pain relief. The PPP Assessment becomes your compass. Your Personal Pain Paradigm carves out your daily passage. The biweekly newsletter from www.MyPainReliefDoc.com is your trusted companion. You have access to everything you need to achieve pain relief. The next step is yours. What do you choose?

APPENDIX

Rhiannon's Sorrow aka Rhia's Resurrection

In the time-honored tradition of passing spoken stories down through generations, I have taken small liberties with this tale, agreeing that, "an' as it harms none, do as ye' will."

Long, long ago there lived King Pwyll who ruled the castle, town, and forest of Dyfed. The dense forest was the home of the mysterious fairy people. Pwyll alone among the human folk was not afraid of the fairies, and one night in the forest came upon the beautiful fairy, Rhiannon, dressed in gold upon a white steed. Professing his love, he asked her to marry, but she commanded that he wait a year to test his love.

A year passed, and when King Pwyll returned to the forest, Rhiannon agreed to marry him and live in his castle. The people were distrusting of the fairy queen, but her goodness won them over. Eventually, she bore the king a beautiful son and everyone rejoiced in the new heir to the throne.

One night, as Rhiannon slept, her infant disappeared right under the sleeping noses of the women who were guarding him. The women discovered the disappearance and, in fear for their lives, they decided to accuse the queen of murdering her own son. They smeared deer's blood on the sleeping queen and in the morning dragged her before the king and his counselors with their tale of murder. The counselors were suspicious of fairies anyway and the people turned viciously against the queen, which persuaded the reluctant king to punish her according to custom.

Rhiannon was forced to stand all day outside the castle gates for seven years wearing a heavy, cruel horse collar that was yoked to a carriage. She was made to announce her crime to all passers by. She was forced to pull the king's visitors to him by carriage, which ripped her flesh and nearly bent her in half.

The townspeople abused her terribly for sport. Grief stricken over her child, torn from her home, publicly shamed, and in terrible physical pain, she bore her suffering with courage and dignity. She was kind and respectful to all, no matter how she was treated. Her fairy goodness and light shone through, and as years passed, the people began to feel sorry for her. She became a symbol of integrity despite injustice. The curious and the hopeless traveled far and wide to experience her inner strength and grace.

One day a married couple appeared before Rhiannon with a beautiful, golden haired boy. As they approached, the boy held out a piece of brocaded cloth. Rhiannon gasped because she knew that she had made that cloth. When she looked in the boy's eyes, she knew instantly that he was her son and she hugged him fiercely. "How is this possible?" she cried.

The husband told her that a demon had come to their home to steal a horse, and in the ensuing struggle, had dropped the golden haired infant he was carrying before he fled. The couple had raised the infant as their own, but upon hearing of Rhiannon's tragedy and heroic suffering, they brought the boy home to his mother.

The couple, the boy, and his mother all raced to the castle to tell the king what had happened. But, as soon as he saw his son, he too knew. He wept, embraced his wife, and on his knees begged her forgiveness. She did indeed forgive him and the king and queen allowed the couple to live in the castle with them as trusted advisors and mentors to their son.

The years spent with the collar ferrying travelers to the king had taken their toll. Rhiannon was stooped, her sleep was fitful, and her body ached always. But she had learned that acceptance made all things possible, that hope was more powerful than misery or mistreatment. Her courage, integrity, and grace through suffering had melted the cold hearts of her people, won back a kingdom, and triggered her son's return. And they all lived happily ever after, more days than not.

Bibliography

Aaslip, Elisabeth, *Healing Muscle Pain: Tools, Techniques, and Tips to Bring Your Muscles Back to Health, Wiley: New York, 2001.*

Abelson, Brian, Release Your Pain, Rowan Tree Books Ltd: Calgary, Canada, 2003.

Adams, Rex, *Miracle Medicine Foods*, Reward Books: E. Rutherford, 1977.

Altemus, Barbara, *The Gift of Pain: Transforming Hurt into Healing*, Perigee Books: New York, 2003.

Anderson, William R. and Taylor, Jesse F., Chronic Pain: Taking Command of our Healing: Understanding the Emotional Trauma Underlying Chronic Pain, New Energy Press, Minneapolis, 1995.

Bacci, Ingrid Lorch, *Effortless Pain Relief: A Guide to Self Healing from Chronic Pain*, Free Press: Riverside, 2005.

Bandura, Albert, *Social Learning Theory*, Prentice-Hall, Inc.: Englewood Cliffs, 1977.

Catalano, Ellen M. and Hardin, Kimeron, N, *The Chronic Pain Control Workbook: A Step by Step Guide for Coping with and Overcoming Pain*, Second Edition, New Habinger Publications: Oakland, 1996.

Caudill, Margaret A, *Managing Pain Before It Manages You*, The Guilford Press: New York, 1995.

Davies, Clair, *The Trigger Point Therapy Workbook: Your Self Treatment Guide for pain Relief*, Second Edition, New Harbinger Publications: Oakland, 2004.

Diamond, Seymour, *Conquering Your Migraine, The Essential Guide to Understanding and Treating Migraines for All Sufferers and Their Families*, Fireside: London, 2001.

Dillard, James and Hirschman, Leigh Ann, *The Chronic Pain Solution: Your Personal Path to Pain Relief*, Bantam: New York, 2003.

Egoscue, Pete, *Pain Free: A Revolutionary New Method for Stopping Chronic Pain*, Bantam: New York, 2000.

Ellis, Albert and Harper, Robert, *A Guide to Rational Living*, Wilshire Book Company: North Hollywood, 1986.

Fishman, Scott, *The War on Pain*, HarperCollins Publishers: San Jose, 2001.

Frankl, Victor, *Man's Search for Meaning*, Washington Square Press: New York, 1985.

Goldfarb, Sylvia and Waddell, Roberta W., *Relieving Pain Naturally*, Square One Publishers: Garden City Park, 2004.

Greenhalgh, Susan, *Under the Medical Gaze: Facts and Fictions of Chronic Pain*, University of California Press: Berkeley, 2001.

Hall, Hamilton, *A Consultation with the Back Doctor*, McClelland & Stewart: Plattsburgh, 2004.

Hauser, Ross A and Hauser, Marion A, *Prolo Your Fibromyalgia Pain Away! Curing the Disabling Pain of Fibromyalgia with Prolotherapy*, Beulah Land Press: Oak Park, 2000.

Hauser, Ross A and Hauser, Marion A, *Prolo Your Back Pain Away! Curing Chronic Back Pain Away with Prolotherapy*, Beulah Land Press: Oak Park, 2000.

Hochschuler, Stephen, *Treat Your Back Without Surgery: The Best Nonsurgical Alternatives for Eliminating Back and Neck Pain*, Hunter House: Alameda, 2002.

Jamison, Robert N, *Learning to Master Your Chronic Pain*, Professional Resource Press: Sarasota, 1996.

Key, Sarah, *Back Sufferer's Bible*, Unwin Hyman: New York, 2001.

Marcus, Norman J, and Atbeiter, Jean S., *Freedom from Chronic Pain: The Breakthrough Method of Pain Relief Based on the New York Pain Treatment Program at Lenox Hill Hospital*, Fireside: London, 1995.

McKenzie, Robin and Kubey, Craig, 7 Steps to a Pain Free Life: How to Rapidly Relieve Back and Neck Pain, Plume Books: New York, 2001.

McIlwain, Harris H. and Bruce, Debra Fulghum, *The Pain-Free Back: 6 Simple Steps to End Pain and Reclaim Your Life*, Owl Books: Toronto, 2004.

Melzack, Ronald and Wall, Patrick, *The Challenge of Pain*, Penguin Global: New York, 1999.

Moskowitz, Peter and Lang, Linda, *Living with RSDS: Your Guide to Coping With Reflex Sympathetic Dystrophy Syndrome*, New Harbinger Publications: Oakland, 2003.

Pinsky, Drew, *When Painkillers Become Dangerous: What Everyone Needs to know about OxyContin and Other Prescription Drugs*, Hazelden: Center City, 2004.

Prudden, Bonnie, *Pain Erasure: The Bonnie Prudden Way*, Ballantine Books: Westminster, 2002.

Puotinen, C.J., *Natural Relief from Aches and Pains*, McGraw-Hill Companies: New York, 2001.

Rapoport, Alan M. and Sheftell, Fred D., *Headache Relief for Women: How You Can Manage and Prevent Pain*, Little, Brown: New York, 1996.

Robinson, Lynne, *The Pilates Prescription for Back Pain: A Comprehensive Program for Developing and Maintaining a Healthy Back*, Ulysses Press: Berkeley, 2004.

Rome, Jeffrey. *Mayo Clinic on Chronic Pain*, Kensington Publishing Corporation: Kalamazoo, 2002.

Ronald, M., *Magnet Therapy: The Pain Cure Alternative*, Prima Lifestyles: New York, 1998.

Rosenfeld, Arthur, *The Truth About Chronic Pain*, Basic Books: New York, 2003.

Rutstein, Joel E, *Take Back Control of Your Arthritis: The 12 Critical Steps*, Xlibris Corporation: Philadelphia, 2004.

Sarno, John, *Freedom from Fibromyalgia: The 5-week Program Proven to Conquer Pain*, 1st edition, Three Rivers Press: Three Rivers, 2001.

Sarno, John, *Mind Over Back Pain: A Radically New Approach to the Diagnosis and Treatment of Back Pain*, Berkeley Publishing Group: Berkeley, 1999.

Sarno, John, *Healing Back Pain: The Mind Body Connection*, Warner Books: London, 1991.

Schatz, Mary P, *Back Care Basics: A Doctor's Gentle Yoga Program for Back and Neck Pain Relief*, Rodmell Press: Berkeley, 1992.

Schneider, Jennifer, *Living with Chronic Pain: The Complete Health Guide to the Causes and Treatment of Chronic Pain*, Healthy Living Books: Traverse City, 2004.

Shapiro, David, *Neurotic Styles*, Basic Books: New York, 1965.

Silver, Julie K., *Chronic Pain and the Family: A New Guide*, (The Harvard University Press Family Health Guides), 2004.

Sinel, Michael S. and Deardorff, William W., *Back Pain for Dummies*, For Dummies: Hoboken, 1999.

Skinner, B.F., *About Behaviorism*, Random House: New York, 1976.

Stauth, Cameron and Khalsa, Dharma Singh, *The Pain Cure: The Proven Medical Program that Helps End Your Chronic Pain*, Warner Books: London, 1999.

Weller, Stella, *The Yoga Back Book*, Thorsons Publishers: London, 2000.

Wolpe J. and Lazarus, A., *Behavior Therapy Techniques*, Pergamon Press: Oxford, 1966.

References

Alvarez, David J, and Rockwell, Pamela G, *American Family Physician*, 2002; Vol. 65/No.4.

Bernstein, Clifford, personal communication, 2005.

Burns, David D., *Feeling Good: The New Mood Therapy*, Avon Books: New York, 1979.

Cameron, Sandy, personal communication, 2005.

Gurskis, John, personal communication, 1994.

Hanson, Richard W. and Gerber, Kenneth E., *Coping With Chronic Pain*, Guilford Press: New York, 1990.

Helm, Standiford II, *Pain Physician*, 2004; Vol. 7, pp 229-238.

Hess, Carl, personal communication, 2005.

Manchikanti, L, Kloth D, Singh V, et al., *Pain Physician*, 2003; Vol. 6, pp 3-81.

Merritt, Andrew, personal communication, 2005.

Paicius, Richard, personal communication, 2005.

Price, D.D., et al. In Fields, H.L. and Liebeskind, J.C., eds. *Pharmacological approaches to the Treatment of Chronic Pain: New concepts and Critical Issues*, IASP Press, Seattle, 1994:66.

Sata, Holly, personal communication, 2004.

Index

978-0-595-38280-4
0-595-38280-0

CPSIA information can be obtained at www.ICGtesting.com
Printed in the USA
LVOW12s2000091214

418025LV00003B/9/P